How to Get the

HEALTH CARE

You Want

THE SAVVY CONSUMER'S GUIDE TO NAVIGATING
THE HEALTH CARE SYSTEM

Laura L. Casey

1 LIFE PRESS

Notice: This book is not intended to replace recommendations or advice from physicians or other health care providers. Rather, it is intended to help you make informed decsions about your health and to cooperate with your health care provider in a joint quest for optimal wellness. If you suspect you have a medical problem, we urge you to seek medical attention from a competent health care provider.

Published by 1 Life Press
P.O. Box 26644, Austin, Texas 78755
www.1lifepress.com

Copyright ©2007 Laura Casey

Distributed by Greenleaf Book Group LP

For ordering information or special discounts for bulk purchases, please contact Greenleaf Book Group LP at 4425 Mopac South, Suite 600, Longhorn Building, 3rd Floor, Austin, TX 78735, (512) 891-6100

Page design, cover, and composition by Greenleaf Book Group LP

Publisher's Cataloging-In-Publication Data
Casey, Laura L.
    How to get the health care you want : the savvy consumer's guide to navigating the health care system / Laura L. Casey. -- 1st ed.

    p. ; cm.
Includes index.

ISBN-13: 978-0-9790730-0-7
ISBN-10: 0-9790730-0-6

1. Medical care—United States—Popular works. 2. Medical personnel and patient—Popular works. 3. Patient education--Popular works. 4. Consumer education—Popular works. 5. Patient satisfaction—Popular works. I. Title.
R727.3 C37 2007
610.69/6 2006937734

Printed in the United States of America on acid-free paper

07 08 09 10 11 12 13   10 9 8 7 6 5 4 3 2 1

First Edition

For Mom

Contents

Introduction

I am a person just like you. When my body doesn't operate as planned, I experience a myriad of reactions, ranging from little or no annoyance to full-blown panic and fear—just like you. *How to Get the Health Care You Want* is a hands-on guide to assist you with managing your care experiences as you navigate our health care system.

Good care is alive and well in our health care delivery system. However, sometimes it may be challenging to find. In this book I will bring to light the signs and symptoms of a variety of care service levels. I will help you navigate those situations so you can find care that meets your personal values, standards, and budget.

In this book you will learn how to create and communicate your expectations to caregivers, how to identify and navigate inappropriate situations relating to customer service and clinical care, and how to better understand the cost of care and your health insurance. At no point in this book am I suggesting that you alter care or treatment plans without the guidance of a physician, nor am I ever implying or suggesting you should forgo care. The goal of this book is to help you have the confidence and ability to craft the care experience that best suits you.

In 1997, my mother was living in Naperville, Illinois, and working as a human resource director for an organization with over five hundred employees. As the cold Chicago winter softened into spring, Mom didn't seem herself. She missed deadlines at work, slept too much, and was forgetful.

My job at the time was taking me to Clinton, Iowa, on a regular basis. Clinton is about a two-hour drive from Naperville. Serendipitously, I was interacting with Mom more than I would have otherwise, as I lived in Vermont. As the spring warmed into summer, her forgetfulness worsened and her personality seemed different. She was diabetic and managed her insulin levels with oral medication. Based on her altered behavior, I thought possibly a switch to insulin injections might be needed. I began asking her to see her physician to find out if in fact a change might be appropriate. She visited her primary care physician, where she had a physical and a sugar test.

Weeks went by and I kept asking her about the results. She hadn't received them, nor did she seem the least bit concerned about her condition or the lack of contact from her doctor's office. Other symptoms were appearing. She had frequent bouts of nausea, while the sleepiness and forgetfulness worsened.

It was hard to intrude into my mother's life as she had made it through fifty-eight years without my help, but I was perplexed. Why, all of a sudden, was she unable to handle this situation? In August I spent a week with her in Naperville, and to my amazement, Mom was no longer Mom. Her ability to manage her day-to-day life was diminishing while her apathy grew. We booked an appointment with her primary care physician.

With no understanding as to what was wrong with Mom, I took on the role of private investigator. I began to analyze her behavior. I read about diabetes and how sugar levels affect a person's demeanor. I gained clear understanding of her medications while soliciting assistance and attention from every health care provider we encountered. I had begun researching Alzheimer's disease.

When we visited her primary care physician's office, she was examined by an intern, not a medical doctor (M.D.), as I had expected. I indicated that Mom really wasn't herself. I told the intern she was forgetful, very sleepy, and experiencing bouts of nausea and vomiting on a regular basis. None of this behavior or physical condition was normal for her.

I indicated she had had a blood sugar test weeks ago and we were still awaiting the results. The intern had the results sitting on his lap in Mom's chart. He said her sugar levels were normal. He also determined that there was nothing wrong with her because she passed a basic neurological exam. The test seemed to focus on analysis of data and numbers: count backward, add a list of numbers together, and follow the light on the end of a pen. Mom performed these tasks flawlessly. I became more baffled.

As more time passed, I became a staple at all of Mom's health-related appointments. At every opportunity I told every clinician we encountered, "Mom is not quite herself; she is forgetful, sleepy, and has frequent bouts of nausea." I was dismissed at every encounter.

Concurrently, Mom was being treated for breast cancer. She had experienced a right breast lumpectomy four years prior. She was now experiencing an abnormality with her left breast. At this juncture, Mom's ability to grasp her treatment options for the breast cancer was diminished. I called the nurse at the surgeon's office and asked her to revisit the treatment options with Mom on three different occasions. Finally, Mom chose a lumpectomy with radiation. The surgery went well. Forty-eight hours after the surgery, however, her vomiting and nausea escalated.

As you might begin to imagine, the weeks of research, reaching out to health care providers to no avail, and the degradation of Mom's condition and behavior brought my frustration to new personal levels. At 11:00 on a Friday night in early September, just forty-eight hours after Mom's breast surgery, her vomiting continued. I called her health insurance plan to see what we could do.

The nurse and I won Mom a trip to the emergency room when the nurse asked, "So she hasn't had fluids stay down for over seventeen hours?" I had no recollection how many hours had elapsed, but *yes* was my answer. The nurse said we could head to the hospital.

We arrived at the local ER at approximately 11:30 p.m. and sat down at check-in. Along with indicating Mom's recent breast surgery, I again stated, "Mom is not herself; she is sleepy, forgetful, and nauseous." When

Mom completed the admissions form, she answered the insurance question "relationship to subscriber" with "Daughter." Mom, the savvy human resource director, who maintained a thorough understanding of health insurance and health plans as part of her job, answered *daughter*! How could she not know the correct answer was herself?

I pointed to the response on the intake form and asked the admitting representative to note that the incorrect response was highly irregular for Mom, and to please point the inappropriate response out to the doctor. The representative indicated he would pass the comment along to the doctor.

Once in an exam room, a nurse began taking down Mom's history, vital signs, and so on. The nurse turned to me and asked, "Is this normal for her?" I responded with an enormously relieved *no*. Finally, someone was going to hear me and believe me. Finally, someone noticed. Finally, someone *cared*.

My moment of relief was quickly dashed when the ER physician entered the room. He routinely examined Mom and determined that she should go home with meds for an upset stomach and drink lots of fluids. He made no mention of any of the data we had provided both the nurse and the admitting representative.

I restated, "Mom is not herself. She is very sleepy, nauseous, and forgetful, and has been that way for months. Your nurse even noticed it."

The ER doctor replied, "You should go home and take care of your mother."

To this point, after weeks and weeks of describing Mom's altered state to clinician after clinician, not once had I lost my cool. The comment, "Go home and take care of your mother," however, struck a nerve. I responded in desperation, "I *am* taking care of my mother. I live in Vermont, we are all standing here in Illinois, and I can assure you there is something wrong!" He left the room.

During the time alone with Mom, I actually contemplated leaving her there in the ER out of utter frustration and desperation. I wanted to walk out of the hospital and abandon her. The thought entered my mind as a strategy, not a sincere desire to abandon Mom. I wanted to see what they would do with a fifty-eight-year-old woman at 2:00 a.m. who, at a minimum, was dehydrated and had no family member to take her home. I wondered if that was how to force them to care for her. I was showing signs of irrationality.

The ER physician came back and asked questions about her breast cancer. After another fifteen-minute negotiation, he agreed to perform a CT scan of Mom's brain. Despite all her care relating to breast cancer, no one had scanned her brain to see if the breast cancer had traveled there.

At 3:00 a.m. we were looking at what we would learn days later was a 7 × 9 × 2 cm brain tumor. Mom's postoperative pathology report would confirm a grade IV primary brain cancer diagnosis called Glioblastoma Multiforme. This type of cancer had nothing to do with her breast cancer. After months of appointments, words, communication, care, concern, and frustration, Mom finally had everyone's attention.

When we seek care we expect to be cared for every step of the way. We want competent and efficient access with no waiting to receive test results or clinical attention. We expect continuous, clear communication from everyone involved, and we expect everyone to care and contribute positively to our journey as we return to a state of wellness.

Mom had her right frontal lobe removed three days later. She lived four-and-a-half months after the initial tumor was diagnosed and removed, and during that time we found incredible caregivers in Illinois and Vermont. We had a memorable full four-plus months of life. When Mom reached the end of her own life she was bedridden for eight days in the comfort of supportive hospice care and her family.

In addition to living with Mom as she died, life has offered me the experience of living with a spouse in chronic jaw pain for nine years, as well as my own personal healing experiences, which include surgery. The professional side of me focuses on a health care–related career that began in 1987. I work within the financial and insurance arena of billing and collections for physician-oriented organizations. My twenty-year professional career has offered me the opportunity to personally experience hundreds of physician practices of varying specialties throughout the country.

The combination of these personal and professional health care life experiences has brought this guide to fruition. As a fellow consumer of care, I hope to teach you how to find good care that suits your needs, values, expectations, and budget.

1

What Are Your Goals?

— — — — — — — — — — — — — — — — —

Most of us maintain a primary goal to be healthy. When we become unhealthy, regaining our quality of life and health becomes paramount. When we need care, we enter the health care delivery system with the expectation that we will be cared for and healed. We expect health care professionals to fix our ailing body—and fix it in a timely fashion. Generally, the combination of our body's ability to heal and the expertise of our health care professionals creates a positive outcome, and we return to a state of wellness after treatment. Sometimes, however, our journey to that positive outcome wasn't at all what we wanted, asked for, or expected.

When getting well is our priority, we become very active participants in the healing process. Shouldn't we then expect a health care delivery system to meet us with the same focus and intensity? If the goal is to return to *your life*, as quickly as possible, then don't you need to set the stage for what you expect from your health care providers? Don't you then need to communicate those expectations with your health care providers and hold them accountable for your mutually agreed upon expectations? And, if a provider doesn't or can't meet those expectations, then don't you need to find a provider who does agree and is able to meet your expectations? Easier said than done.

Power, according to *Webster's*, is "[the] ability to act or produce effect . . . possession of control authority or influence over others." The power of wellness enables American consumers to command the best of everything this world has to offer. When illness sets in we seem to dismiss our consumer power and leave it in the parking lot of the health care facility. As we cross the threshold of the health care facility we forget that we are at the helm, and we can craft our health care experience in conjunction with our care providers. In the dismissal of our consumer-based power we accept poor systems and mediocrity, and consequently give up our influence and control of our personal goals.

Finding and maintaining your consumer power or assertiveness is difficult and sometimes not possible when you are sick. When you are the patient focused on your healing, you may not be able to advocate on your own behalf. When your situation is such that your illness has taken over and your consumer-oriented power and assertiveness are not accessible, you need to have a healthy person by your side facilitating your return to wellness. This person or advocate will communicate your values and needs to the health care providers and systems, ensuring you receive the care you wish to receive.

Never Hesitate to Advocate

In today's business-oriented, managed care driven climate, finding the family practitioner who services entire families and all their needs, both emotional and physical, across generations is a precious gem. Our systematic business approach to care typically turns the role of advocate over to a family member, friend, or case worker.

Because the nature of such long-term relationships spanning generations with primary care doctors has changed, patients and their family members may find themselves feeling alone, frightened, and frustrated, particularly when illness is serious or life threatening. When the role of the clinical communicator, facilitator, and advocate has fallen by the wayside, patients most often look to family members to keep their care on the straight and narrow.

If you are the patient entering the foreign world of a disease, condition, procedure, or trauma, you need support. Utilize a loved one as a patient advocate, and if a loved one is not available, solicit the support of a social worker, clergy, or friend. The role of your personal advocate is to be your eyes, ears, and scribe. This person keeps your care organized in conjunction with your team of medical doctors. They log your questions and their answers, they read your medical record to ensure its accuracy, and if you are unable, they prompt clinical and nonclinical staff for your needs. Additionally, your advocate maintains your personal health record for you until you are able. Communication and trust between all parties is paramount.

Your advocate's role can vary widely, and the person need not be a savvy health care expert. The person does, however, need to confidently assert themselves on your behalf. Your advocate needs to represent and be your consumer power and voice when you are not able. This person is not by your side to dictate your care. This person is by your side to validate or double-check all care-related communication between you and your caregivers. The role can be as mundane as returning your dinner to the hospital kitchen because you ordered applesauce, not fruit cup. Or, the gravity of the responsibility can be serious and critical, like finding you a brain surgeon because you've been diagnosed with brain cancer and have decided surgery is your next step.

After my father's heart surgery, he moved to a room on the cardiac floor of the hospital. The concept of heart surgery was quite frightening for him. Despite the success of the operation, he maintained a high level of anxiety during the initial period following the surgery.

Advocating for a patient is a combination of listening, watching, and feeling. Dad withdrew from the mundane chatter surrounding him. When we noticed he was no longer participating in the conversation, we asked if something was wrong. All he could describe at that moment was that he felt "funny." He said, "My heart feels funny." We all paused to see what our next clue might be.

As the moments ticked by, the tension grew with his fear and anxiety. We didn't wait long to summon a nurse, nor did we use the nurse call button. I exited Dad's room, found a nurse at the nurse's station, and requested she come check him out right then

Within a few minutes, we all understood what Dad's funny feeling was, and the nurse began taking the necessary steps to slow his heart rate down.

In this example, I participated in Dad's care by simply getting him the attention he perceived he needed at that moment. He didn't have to wait and wonder if the call button from his bed was working. He didn't have to live through the funny feeling alone.

Depending on the severity of your condition, the person acting as the advocate may attend all of your clinical appointments and procedures. This person's role is not to tell you what to do or dictate your care to clinicians, but to facilitate any and all mutually agreed upon care steps that you have made with your doctor(s). This person needs to be aware of your wishes and cognizant of everything going on around you during the care experience. Your doctor(s) should know who your advocate is and interact with you both (with your permission).

Should you find yourself in the unexpected role as advocate because the health issue is serious or urgent, let your common sense and intuition prevail. Listen intently, engage all supportive resources available to you, and do your best to hold any irrational emotion at bay during the crisis. Periods of crisis require vigilance, level-headed decision making, and communication. It's not my nature to ask for help during the course of my day-to-day life. However, through my experience with Mom's brain cancer I learned not only that it's okay to ask for help, but also that there are scores of fabulous people who will offer competent and relevant support and assistance during the patient's time of need. Ask for help when you need it.

Once we learned Mom's issue was a brain tumor, we were inundated with information and support because we asked for help. One doctor said don't operate, it's not a cure. Another doctor said the CT scan is just a picture; you must operate because only a specimen can confirm exactly what kind of tumor is present, and the type of tumor will dictate the treatment plan. A friend searched the Internet and faxed to us all sorts of data relating to Mom's brain cancer.

The information was important to us, and we did our best to assimilate it all in a forty-eight-hour period. By the time Mom headed to the operating room for her brain surgery, we were all thoroughly exhausted. She wanted surgery, and we did our best to learn about and find the best and most appropriate care for her. As her advocates, we had done our job.

There are many avenues to pursue in addition to friends and family when you need support. Start with your company's Employee Assistance Program (EAP) if you or a family member is employed. Most EAP services are underutilized, and they are usually free. In general, an EAP program offers research services and counseling support for you and your family, and provides documentation. If you aren't employed, then seek the assistance of your local social services (see chapter 7) or clergy. Depending on the patient's condition, hospice or mental health counseling may be appropriate suggestions for the patient and family members.

2

The Communication Cycle: Our Role as Patients

Communicate, Participate, Evaluate, and Communicate

Never hesitate to advocate and communicate about everything. *Communicate* with your caregivers so they know and understand what hurts, what is important to you, why you are seeking care, how you feel, that you are scared, confident, happy, and that blueberries don't taste good anymore. Whatever you believe is important and pertains to the re-creation of your wellness is important information for you to communicate to your health care providers. What the provider does with that information will tell you whether or not this provider is a match for you. As adult patients navigating a health care delivery system, our role is to communicate as clearly, completely, and honestly as possible.

When interacting with doctors, we assist the healing process by providing as much comprehensive and accurate information as possible. Tell your doctor about your apprehension and concerns. If you stopped taking the medications prescribed at your last visit because they made you dizzy, then say that. If you stopped taking your medications because you can't afford them this month, then say that.

Keep a health journal that tracks not only your actions but also the actions of your caregivers. The stresses of illness can often make us forgetful and more easily confused. Write down your symptoms. Track your health-related experiences, write down your questions and the answers, and then evaluate and note how the provider performed. If you cannot write down your own questions or answers, then request a loved one or patient advocate assist with your documentation. Usually a loved one or family member takes on the role of scribe. If you are alone, ask one of your caregivers to assist with your note taking, or request a case worker from Social Services.

Chapter 5 provides a suggested structure for your health record. Maintain your own data as you travel the road to wellness. Write everything down, or have it written down for you, and be certain you understand the answers to your questions. If you don't understand what is going on, then ask again. If you disagree with your care, most certainly speak your opinion. *Participate* in your care.

Evaluate your caregivers. Caregivers expand far beyond the doctor and the nurse, so clear, direct communication is important through every stage of your care process. When a nurse's aid dumped a full bag of urine from my foley catheter all over me and my bed the day after I had my kidney removed, you might imagine it was a mess I really didn't need at that moment in my life. I was twenty-one, and even at that age I told my surgeon, "I never want to see her (the nurse's aid) again." I told my surgeon that particular nurse's aid was incompetent, and her inability to care for me was unacceptable. Consequently, I never saw her again. Poor performers will add stress to your healing experience. It's important to communicate and remove the poor performers from your care experience.

Don't leave or allow the caregiver to leave until all of your questions have been answered satisfactorily. You should be in agreement with the treatment plan and have a means to obtain support and get future questions answered on off hours should they arise. Be certain you have a feeling of comfort and reassurance from your visit. Participate in your care.

Communicate, participate, evaluate, and *communicate* with each individual you encounter while on the road to wellness. Even though you may not feel well, get organized or get someone to get you organized. If you are unorganized the otherwise minor issues or unexpected bumps in the road will feel enormous or block the path entirely. The more complex or chronic the illness, the more care needed, and therefore the more organized you need to be in order to reduce the potential stressors related to the imperfections of the health care delivery system.

Heightened organization on your part will also offer more efficiency as you navigate your care experience. If your body is not functioning 100 percent and your quality of life is lacking, what becomes your focus? Wellness. If you had the choice to become well in thirty seconds or thirty days, most of us would choose thirty seconds. Who wants to spend time in pain, feel run down, or bothered by a runny nose for a month? When we are seeking health and wellness, time matters.

If you were a person with grade IV brain cancer, which means there is no cure, you are going to die soon, and you know it, and your radiation oncologist (cancer doctor) created a standing order (a prescription that automatically repeats and is meant to be used again and again at a particular time interval) for weekly blood work, and each Tuesday you headed to the lab after your radiation treatment, as ordered, to have your blood drawn, would you really want to be told by the lab staff week after week that you have to go downstairs and register with admissions again? Would you really want to spend twenty minutes of your life every week repeating a clerical task that adds no value to your quality of life when you know you are dying?

For those of us who don't have the luxury of knowing we're going to die soon, the redundant request to register for lab work every week may be perceived merely as a nuisance. If, however, you know you are going to die, soon, or you know the person standing next to you is going to die soon, the request to spend the time on a redundant task that adds no benefit to the healing, wellness, or quality of life becomes a ridiculous and unacceptable request.

Aren't we *all* going to die soon? Navigating a health care system that requires taking repetitive steps that waste our time, detracts from our lifetime, and insults our physical body repeatedly or unnecessarily due to incompetence and poorly designed systems is unacceptable. As patients, we select our treatment paths. The health care provider's role is to facilitate the process in conjunction with our communicated values, goals, and expectations.

A friend needed a pacemaker. Millions of people have pacemakers, so the procedure to get a pacemaker in today's world, if common sense were to prevail, certainly must be well defined. My friend got his pacemaker, and life was good. Several months later his pacemaker was recalled. Understandably, he didn't want to be walking around with a faulty pacemaker, so he scheduled an appointment to receive a new one.

Very soon after receiving the new pacemaker, it became evident something was wrong. Apparently they, whoever *they* are, "forgot" to connect one of the wires. The procedure was repeated so the wire could be connected. My friend had no issue with the fact the initial pacemaker had a recall. Quite rationally, he realized his pacemaker was a device, and like any other device, it could have malfunctions. He didn't mind having it replaced—one time. When he learned "they forgot to plug me in," as he refers to it, the entire experience changed and negatively affected his life.

He became untrusting and fearful of both the device and the people who were supposed to care for him. It took months for him to feel comfortable and believe the new pacemaker would work properly. He had this nagging thought, "What if it becomes unplugged?" Most importantly, he felt as though no one cared. No one cared enough to get it right the first time. No one cared that his body was invaded one time more than it had to be. No one cared about his frustration, anger, and skepticism. No one cared about how much of his lifetime was wasted because of the carelessness of others.

Providers and systems that *care* surely wouldn't purposefully burden us by wasting our time. Providers and systems that care wouldn't offer incorrect information or omit important information or disregard incompetence. Providers and systems that care work with us, understand us, communicate with us, and seek to create mutually agreed upon treatment paths based on our lives and our choices. Then, they execute the treatment paths with a level of competency that is able to navigate the unexpected and recognize that an unexpected deviation from the treatment path will affect you in unexpected ways.

Creating Your List of Standard Care Expectations

Create your list of standard care expectations. The list will apply to almost every health care–related visit you have, and you can always add to it. Know and follow your plans and expectations, and always make a point to communicate those plans and expectations to the caregiver each step of the way. Use the chart in exhibit 2-1 as a guideline for structuring your own list of standard care expectations. Give some thought as to what is important to you when you are dealing with health care providers.

Based on your evaluation of the entire encounter, consciously decide whether you will continue to seek care from the doctor or facility again. Do the people and their processes meet your needs, values, and budget?

There are no right and wrong answers when you reach the evaluation phase. If you communicate and participate throughout the care process and pay close attention to your emotions, the conclusions you need to draw at the evaluation stage will be clear. Competent caring individuals and systems will diminish anxiety. As responsible patients, we must complete the communication cycle. Be sure to convey your evaluation to your health care provider, offering compliments and suggestions where needed.

EXHIBIT 2-1 STANDARD CARE EXPECTATIONS

PERSONAL PREFERENCES

1. Care means _____ to me.
2. I am seeking care because, _____.
3. I believe _____ will cure me.
4. List life stressors that may be contributing to this illness: (for example)

My job	My parent
My marriage	Loss of loved one
My divorce	Loss of job
My child	Abusive relationship
My home	Drug or alcohol abuse

5. To what level or degree do I want to participate in the decision-making process of my care?
6. I want a male/female doctor.
7. I care/don't care about the physician's primary language.
8. I want my doctor to have been in practice _____ years.
9. I need this doctor to integrate with a team of doctors already working on my issue. I will bring the care team's contact sheet with me to this visit.
10. I need to communicate my expectation that the team communicate well among itself.
11. List the team members and their contact information.
12. I expect my clinician to be an M.D., PA, intern, etc. (See chapter 4 definitions.)

ACCESS

1. I expect to be seen in _____ hours/days/weeks/months.
2. I expect the appointment booking process to take less than _____ minutes/hours/days/months.
3. I expect to wait no more than _____ minutes/hours/days/weeks for my health care service.
4. I expect to describe my symptoms or tell my story to no more than _____ person(s).
5. I have prepared a health record for this illness/exam and will share it with my doctor in a written format. (See chapter 5.)
6. I expect to provide my personal and insurance information to no more than _____ person(s). I will bring my personal medical record and family history in written form to all appointments when I am meeting with a new doctor.
7. I expect to pay _____ dollars for this service.

Ask questions 8 and 9 before and after your visit.

8. My tolerance for redundancies and inefficiencies is 0 1 2 3 4 5 6 7 8 9 10 (0 being not at all tolerant and 10 being extremely tolerant).

9. My tolerance for timeliness is 0 1 2 3 4 5 6 7 8 9 10 (0 being not at all tolerant and 10 being extremely tolerant).

10. I expect to spend _____ hours/days/weeks/months/lifetime healing this health issue, or I will ask my doctor how long I should expect to spend healing this issue.

EVALUATE

Apprehension Index
How much anxiety is this health care encounter causing? This is a measure not of the anxiety caused by the illness but of the increase or decrease in anxiety related to the general level of care received.

    1 = no anxiety
    2 = mild anxiousness/annoyance
    3 = apprehension/anger
    4 = fearfulness/rage
    5 = panic and fear/irrationality

Assess your emotional state or the emotional state of the patient for whom you are advocating: Did the encounter create more or less emotion? Did your fear, anxiety, and anger levels rise or fall? Was stress encountered? What was its source? Did it relate to your illness or results, or was it related to an incompetent person, a poor communicator, unclean facility, or an inefficient process? Did everyone do what they said they were going to do? No more, no less? Was your care experience positive? Are you stressed due to your illness or due to an incompetent receptionist or a long wait for test results? Does a question nag at you all night because you have no means to seek an answer?

If fear, anxiety, and anger are present during your health care encounter, use the emotional reaction as a tool to evaluate your experience. Understand you may experience fear, anxiety, and anger because of your illness, but do your best to evaluate your emotions as they relate to the people or processes you encountered. Generally, poor systems and incompetent people will cause your stress level relating to the encounter or appointment to rise because you may feel unsafe or insecure. Conversely, good systems and caring, competent people will put you at ease and your anxiety will remain neutral or diminish.

How to Organize Your Care Concerns

If we follow the simple structure of a SOAP note, your thoughts and questions will be handy, organized, and comprehensive.

- **Subjective**, or what is important and relevant positive and negative information. This information could be your history or a description of what is currently going on with your body and life. In other words, tell your story.

- **Objective**, or important findings. This includes data such as test results or physical statistics.

- **Assessment**, or a priority listing of what you believe is wrong—in other words, your diagnosis. What do you feel needs attention? How is your life affected, and what are your priorities?

- **Plan**, or determine what's next. What are your questions, concerns, and criticisms? What is your ideal treatment path? How does this problem get resolved?[1]

SCENARIO 1: A PERSONAL PLAN

My chief complaint for this visit is the head and chest cold that began five days ago. It has not improved since we created a treatment plan. My stomach pain and hives are new as of today.

S: What do you need to tell the caregiver(s)? Give them positive and negative thoughts, feelings, signs, and symptoms. Tell the story.

1. I stopped taking the antibiotics because I had awful stomach pain on Wednesday night, and I got no sleep.
2. I am still wheezing and coughing, and now have hives all over my body.
3. I have new insurance and I have a new card because I got a new job last month. My new insurance went into effect on Monday.

O: What are the important and relevant physical changes since your last visit? Bring your lab test results.

1. I lost three pounds.
2. I still have a sore throat. Is it strep?
3. I itch all over.

A: What do you believe is wrong? What do you feel needs attention? How is your life affected, and what are your priorities?

1. I want the itching and the hives addressed immediately.
2. I want to be able to sleep.
3. What causes hives?
4. I've scratched at the hives. Is that bad?
5. What was the name of the antibiotic that gave me the severe stomach pain? Did it cause my hives?
6. How do I know new or different antibiotics will not cause my stomach to hurt again?
7. If I encounter Nurse Tom, I will give him another opportunity, and I will *evaluate* his attentiveness.

P: What is your plan? What are your questions, concerns, and criticisms? What is your ideal treatment path? How does this problem get resolved?

1. They were supposed to correct my bill; I need to check that, too.
2. Last time they made me wait twenty-five minutes in the waiting room and another twenty minutes in the exam room. This lengthy wait is outside my tolerance for waiting and is unacceptable. I am going to tell the doctor I will seek a new provider once I am well and the reason for the change is that I wait too long to be seen.

My standard care questions and plan assessment are

1. Do I really need the care they are proposing?

2. Do I really need the medications they are prescribing?

3. Will this treatment plan enhance my quality of life and wellness?

4. How do I expect this plan to enhance my life and wellness?

SCENARIO 2: AN ADVOCATE'S PLAN

My chief complaint for this visit is that Mom just had nodules removed from her throat. The lab report indicates cancer. This is my first visit to the oncologist with Mom.

S: What do you need to tell the caregiver(s)? Give them positive and negative thoughts, feelings, signs, and symptoms. Tell the story.

1. Mom is very emotional. She cries most of the day. She is afraid she is going to die.

2. She can't eat normally because she is sore from the surgery. When can she expect to eat normally?

3. She wants to know what is wrong with her body immediately.

O: What are the important and relevant physical changes since your last visit to this caregiver? Bring your lab test results.

1. Considerable swelling continues since the drains were removed after her surgery.

2. The lab is supposed to send the lab results to the oncologist (better call to double-check).

3. The radiologist is supposed to send all of Mom's films and reports to the oncologist (call to check that they arrived).

4. I have and will bring Mom's health records.

A: What do you believe is wrong? What do you feel needs attention? How is your life affected, and what are you priorities?

1. Does Mom like the doctor?

2. Is she and her staff caring?

3. Are the patients who are clearly dying in plain view of those who are not?

P: What is your plan? What are your questions, concerns, and criticisms? What is your ideal treatment path? How does this problem get resolved?

1. Finish calling references for the oncologist.

2. Search the Internet for more information pertaining to Mom's alleged cancer.

3. Listen and take notes during Mom's visit.

4. Bring Mom's medical record, including the list of medications.

5. What treatment is recommended, and why?

6. Where will the treatment occur?

7. How will the treatment occur, and how often?

8. Is this proposed treatment a new treatment?

9. What are other treatment options?

10. Is this treatment covered by her insurance?

11. What are the benefits of this treatment?

12. What are the risks to have the treatment?

13. What are the risks to not have this treatment?

14. What medicine or chemotherapy will she be given?

15. What side effects will she have?

16. Will she experience hair loss? Where can I get a wig for her? Will insurance pay for it?

17. Do you have information we can read?

18. How do I reach you during off hours? What is your twenty-four-hour support like?

19. I have Mom's referral form for the oncologist, and it has been filed with her insurance. What other insurance-related tasks do I need to complete?

20. I have her insurance card and will bring it.

21. Can she be left alone?

22. Will she need more surgery?

23. Search the Internet for credentials and complaints lodged for all care-givers.

At this time, Mom is too emotional to answer the questions relating to her standard care expectations. Once we get some of my questions answered, I hope to have her communicate her standards to me.

SCENARIO 3: A PERSONAL PLAN FOR SURGERY

My chief complaint for this visit is that I am twenty-one years old and have a nonfunctioning kidney that must be removed.

S: What do you need to tell the caregiver(s)? Give them positive and negative thoughts, feelings, signs, and symptoms. Tell the story.

1. I am scared and angry.

2. What does all of this mean to my life?

3. What is going to happen to me?

O: What are the important and relevant physical changes since your last visit to this caregiver? Bring your lab test results.

1. My fever has lifted.

2. The pain in my right side has gone away.

3. There is no more burning sensation when I urinate.

4. I have my records to bring with me, and I have prepared a self-medical record in written form.

A: What do you believe is wrong? What do you feel needs attention? How is your life affected, and what are you priorities?

1. Are the professionals competent? (second opinion needed)

2. Will the health care providers show proper compassion?
3. Who will actually perform the surgery?
4. Who will assist?
5. What is the recovery period?
6. What are the possible complications?

P: What is your plan? What are your questions, concerns, and criticisms? What is your ideal treatment path? How does this problem get resolved?

1. Get a second opinion.
2. Choose a surgeon.
   a. How many times have you performed this exact operation?
   b. Will you be using any new devices or equipment that you are unfamiliar or less familiar with?
   c. How do I specify you and only you (my surgeon) will perform this surgery?
   d. Are you a board-certified physician? (See chapter 7 for definitions.)
   e. Have you ever had your hospital privileges revoked?
   f. Have you ever been professionally disciplined?

3. Have surgery.
   a. What exactly will they do to my body?
   b. Will it hurt? How much?
   c. Will I vomit from the surgery?
   d. How long will the surgery take?

4. Determine what to expect after surgery.
   a. Will I need dialysis?
   b. How will this affect my life?
   c. Can I still exercise afterward?

d. How much school will I miss?

e. What about my other kidney; is it okay?

f. Why did this kidney stop functioning?

g. How long will I be in the hospital?

h. What if I don't have this surgery?

i. How much will it cost? What if I can't afford to pay?

j. Can you have three people my age and health status contact me regarding their experience with this surgery?

k. What complications might arise?

l. What are the risks?

m. How will I feel for the long haul?

When possible, organize your thoughts, feelings, and questions before you enter a health-related encounter.

3

Access: "Hold, Please"

---

*Every minute spent unfocused on care to restore your health and
quality of life is a wasted moment of your life.*

My car indicated it needed an oil service. I called the dealership to make
the appointment. When I reached the service department, I asked for an
appointment. We agreed upon Tuesday, and then I gave the gentleman on
the other end of the line a list of items in need of attention. In addition to the
oil service, my clutch was making a squeaky noise every time I depressed the
pedal; my air conditioner, when on high, was so loud you couldn't hold a conversation in the car; one of the temperature gauge buttons had broken; and
the top to the ashtray snapped off (despite the fact I am a nonsmoker and
had never used it). Also, the car needed to be detailed, and I needed a loaner
car. The service advisor said, "Great, we will see you Tuesday morning."

I pulled into the service area on Tuesday morning. A smiling woman
directed me as to where to park my car, my license plate told her who I
was, and as soon as I opened the door she greeted me with a genuine,
"Good morning, Ms. Casey, let me take to you to Dave, your service advisor. Would you like some coffee?"

I sat down at Dave's work area, which was outfitted with a phone, computer, and a chair for each of us. This was my third trip to the dealership in three years, and, consequently, my third trip to meet Dave. He greeted me with a smile and said, "Good morning, Laura, how are you?" He then went on to list every single item I had mentioned to the person who booked my appointment.

Dave said, "I see you are here for an oil service, but you've got some other concerns. The clutch is making a noise, your air conditioner is too loud, the ashtray is broken as well as one of the temperature control buttons, and—great, I see you have a coupon for a day at the spa for the detail." We chatted briefly about the clutch and the air conditioner noise and he said, "Okay, let's get you in the loaner car and get you out of here." A quick copy was made of my driver's license and insurance card, and Dave walked me to my loaner car. I was on my way to work in twelve minutes.

The service department at a car dealership is capable of providing my car access to service in a timely fashion. They cared enough to figure out how to know who I was the moment I entered their organization, and they cared enough to be efficient and remember my requests to the letter. As the items on my repair list were attended to, Dave called me to explain what was needed and provided me with the cost for each item.

I kept the loaner until my car was ready two days later. When I picked up my car, I knew what the cost for the repairs would be, the car was ready upon my arrival to the dealership as Dave said it would be, and with the exception that all the temperature read-outs were inadvertently changed to Celsius, the staff at the dealership did what they said they would do.

If a car dealership can figure out how to provide me with what I consider to be superior customer service and excellent communication, why does an average nonurgent health care encounter resemble the following situation?

You call your doctor's office and hear, "Dr. Smith's office, please hold." Not a great way to begin, especially if you have to wait three minutes to speak to the receptionist. The receptionist returns to your call, you state you twisted your ankle at your son's Little League game and need an appointment. You have been to Dr. Smith's office before and as an established patient, you are offered an appointment the next day. You press the receptionist for an appointment today because your ankle is very tender and swollen. She indicates she can squeeze you in at 2:30 that afternoon. That time works for you, because you don't need to get Sandy, your daughter, from soccer practice until 4:30.

You arrive for your appointment at 2:26 p.m. and are greeted by a receptionist who is sequestered behind a glass window. She is on the phone, isn't smiling, and doesn't introduce herself. She hands you a clipboard of paperwork and a pen, and points to another clipboard. "Sign in," she says, phone still pressed to her ear, "and I will need a copy of your insurance card." You comply with all of her requests and take a seat to complete your paperwork.

You hobble back to the closed window to exchange your paperwork for your insurance card. She glances at you with a mildly annoyed look, never quite making eye contact as she rummages through a stack of charts to locate yours. She says, "Your co-payment is twenty-five dollars." You hand the receptionist your debit card. She answers the phone twice while running your card and hands you the authorization copy. You sign it and hobble back to a seat in the waiting room, exchanging no further words with the receptionist. It's now 2:47.

At 3:05, you hobble back to the reception window, and wait for her to hang up the phone and open the window. "How much longer will the wait be?" you ask. She looks up at a hanging rack of charts and says, "You're next." You hobble back to your seat. At 3:11, a person who appears to be a nurse calls your name out to the entire waiting rooming and you hobble to the exam room.

The apparent nurse, who still hasn't mentioned her name or credentials, appears to notice your gait but makes no mention of it. Upon arrival to the exam room she takes your vital signs and asks why you are here.

You say, "I was at Danny, my son's, Little League game; he plays short-stop. It was the last inning of the tournament game and they were winning by one run but bases were loaded, and the other team's heavy hitter was at bat. It was spine tingling; all the parents were on the edge of their seats! The batter hit a hard ground ball practically into left field, and Danny grabbed it, tagged the runner going to third, threw the ball to first, and got the batter out, game over. We won! In all the winning excitement I was jumping up and down on the bleachers and twisted my ankle. It hurts and is swollen."

The apparent nurse asks, "How long ago did this happened? Have you taken anything for it?"

You respond that the game ended around noon and you have taken two Advil. The nurse jots a note in your chart and says, "Dr. Smith will be right with you." It's now 3:26.

As you await the arrival of Dr. Smith, you recognize the throbbing in your ankle is worsening. Sadness and anger settle in, as you begin to understand that this ankle glitch is going to get in the way of a few upcoming events. However, you try to remain hopeful and console yourself with the thought, "It's not that bad; Dr. Smith will take care of me."

At 3:39, Dr. Smith enters your exam room. He has your chart, and he mentions you indicated to Sally (that must be the apparent nurse's name) that you have injured your ankle. He begins to poke and prod a bit and indicates you need an X-ray, as it might be broken.

You react, "Broken? It can't be broken! I have to take the Cub Scouts camping this weekend, I promised to help the coach get Danny's team ready for the next tournament game, and of course, I need to work tomorrow. You realize Danny's team won today, don't you? They are going to the state championship!"

Politely indifferent, Dr. Smith smiles and congratulates you on behalf of Danny. He hands you a referral form to get your ankle X-rayed and says he will be back in touch when he gets a report from the radiologist. Sally will be back to tell you what to do in the meantime. It's 3:45.

Sally returns with instructions to use ice and Advil, to keep your foot elevated above your heart, and to wear a soft brace until the results of the X-ray are returned. She warns you that if the ankle is broken, excessive walking could make it worse. It's 3:57.

Feeling sad and frustrated, you hobble back to the receptionist station, wondering how you are going to get dinner together. The receptionist is sitting amidst an array of patient charts and is just finishing a call. She notes you need an X-ray and indicates the radiologist's office is downstairs in suite 101. You can walk in and they will see you. Sadly, you take your paperwork and think, "I'll hobble in, and they will see me." It's 3:59.

Care Analysis

Let's take a moment and analyze this encounter so far. I have a personal expectation that the paperwork portion of my care will take five minutes or less and I am comfortable spending that amount of time on that task. I also believe time spent with a clinician who is contributing to my wellness is time well spent.

LOST LIFETIME

The following analysis of the patient's visit to Dr. Smith's office confirms seventy-eight minutes of *lost lifetime*. I consider time spent waiting, performing redundant tasks or any task that does not directly relate to my personal wellness an irrecoverable loss of my lifetime.

Appointment start time:	2:30 p.m.
Completion time:	3:59 p.m.
Total time:	89 minutes
	-6 minutes with Dr. Smith
	-5 minutes (your personal expectation for clerical interactions)
Lost lifetime:	78 minutes

CARE INDEX

How did the encounter affect the patient? Were the people trained to care for this patient able to successfully delivery the care needed? Exhibit 3-1 charts this encounter.

ANXIETY LEVEL

As you step through your health care encounter you can use your changing levels of stress and anxiety to measure how your caregivers are doing.

EXHIBIT 3-1 CARE INDEX: INITIAL CLINICAL INTERACTION

	INTERACTION WITH PATIENT	EFFECT ON STRESS/FEAR	CARE RATING
DR. SMITH'S RECEPTIONIST	Disorganized, unfriendly, and distracted; added to stress; wasted time	Unnecessary annoyance	Poor
APPARENT NURSE (SALLY)	Cold, mechanical, hurried, possibly unqualified	Added fear and stress by saying, "It could get worse if you walk on it," and offering no solution or comfort	Fair
DR. SMITH	Little to no interest in the patient's life or stress level	Added stress by indicating that it might be broken; increased fear with no outlet to diffuse the fear because of indifference to personal circumstances	Fair

If we take a closer look at this encounter we can deduce the patient's level of anxiety probably increased. If we associate points to key episodes of the encounter and graph the cumulative points, we can graph our experience and use it as a tool to evaluate our care experience.

Zero points equates to no anxiety or neutral anxiety. One point is given for general concern or apprehension; two points for anger, frustration, sadness, or fear; three points for rage and strong emotions; and four points for irrational emotion and behavior. As you move through the experience add or subtract the number of points that represent the change in anxiety level for that episode of the care experience.

For example, the reaction associated with the patient's first realization her ankle may be broken could add a point to the anxiety monitor if Dr. Smith doesn't address the response appropriately. If, however, he does address the concern with care, respect, and clear communication and the mild fear is quelled, then the episode would add zero points or possibly subtract points from the accumulated total, because by the end of the interaction the patient's anxiety had been addressed by the caregiver.

EXHIBIT 3-2 INITIAL ANXIETY LEVELS

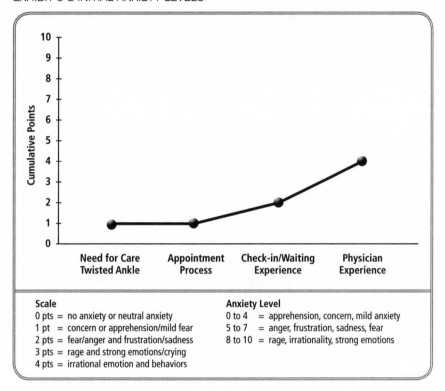

If the experience diminishes stress, then reduce the cumulative points by the difference in points associated with the changed anxiety level. For example, if the interaction changed your feelings from rage to calm relief, then you would subtract two points. The points are quite subjective and only meaningful to you. If you are consistent with your additions and subtractions your graph will depict how you felt throughout the encounter. See exhibit 3-2.

Let's Continue

As you hobble to the radiologist's office, you call your spouse and make arrangements for Sandy to get picked up from soccer practice. You suggest pizza for the kids for dinner, because you don't know when you will get home. You enter the radiologist's office; the waiting area is about half-filled with other patients. It's 4:07.

You present your insurance card and the form from Dr. Smith's receptionist. The radiologist's receptionist hands you a clipboard of forms to be completed, with many of the same questions you just completed for Dr. Smith. She also asks you to sign in on the walk-in log (again you think, "hobble in"). As you turn to take a seat, the receptionist indicates that your insurance requires authorization for diagnostic services, to which you respond, "What does that mean?"

The receptionist states, "You need to get 'auth-ed' before you can be seen."

Your ankle hurts, your ego hurts, you are sad and frustrated, you are missing the postgame celebration, and you have no idea what this woman is talking about. What registers is that the situation just went from bad to worse: You can't get your X-ray taken today, and that means you won't go on the camping trip, and you will miss helping the team prep for the next tournament game. You bark at the receptionist, "What does that *mean*?!"

Your bark is met with an eye roll, your insurance card, and a telephone. The receptionist points to the back of your insurance card and says, "It is the patient's responsibility to get 'auth-ed' for this service. Call this number on your insurance card and answer their questions." It's 4:20.

As you stand on your good leg and lean awkwardly over the reception desk, you call the number on the back of your insurance card. Your frustration is compounded by the thought that you can't even mind the words of Dr. Smith's nurse to keep your ankle elevated. As you look down at your swollen ankle, you feel contempt for the woman behind the desk because she is preventing you from following the prescribed path to wellness per Dr. Smith's office. After a period of hold time, and after answering a myriad of what you perceive to be ridiculous questions, you have been "auth-ed" by the insurance company and can take a seat. It's 4:28.

At 4:41, an X-ray technologist calls your name and you begin to hobble toward her. She notes your discomfort and offers you a wheelchair. As she wheels you to the X-ray machine, she says, "My name is Denise. I am a registered X-ray technologist. What happened?"

You say, "I twisted my ankle at my son's Little League game, and it really hurts."

She responds, "I can see you are in pain. What position does your son play?"

"He plays shortstop. Do you think my ankle is broken?"

Denise responds that she doesn't know if the ankle is broken or not, but she will be sure to take a clear picture for the radiologist so she can see for certain what is going on. "Did your son's team win today?" she asks.

Your response is led with a tiny smile as you recall the winning play of the game. You describe the game to Denise as she takes three pictures of your ankle. As Denise sends you home, she indicates that the results of your X-ray will be sent to Dr. Smith's office by this time tomorrow. You ask Denise if the results can be sent to you directly and as soon as they are ready. Denise indicates she can send you the results, but her office's policy is to send the results to your primary doctor first and then, if you want a copy after you converse with your doctor, she will be happy to send you a copy.

Deflated by the impending twenty-four-hour wait to know what's wrong, you still thank Denise for her care. Denise asks you if you need a cab or would like wheelchair assistance to your car. You feel able to drive, but would welcome a wheelchair ride to your car. It is 5:02; you are on your way home.

Care Analysis

Let's return to our three-point care analysis and evaluate where the patient is at this point.

LOST LIFETIME

Appointment start time:	4:07
Completion time:	5:02
Total time:	55 minutes
	-21 minutes with Denise
	- 5 minutes (personal expectation for clerical interactions)
Lost lifetime:	29 minutes
Cumulative lost lifetime:	107 minutes (1 hour 47 minutes)

(Cumulative lost lifetime is the time spent since the very beginning of the encounter at Dr. Smith's office plus the time spent at the radiologist's office.)

CARE INDEX

Exhibit 3-3 shows the care index at this encounter.

ANXIETY LEVEL

Exhibit 3-4 adds the receptionist and X-ray technologist to the anxiety chart.

You arrive home, and your family greets you. Again, you congratulate Danny for a great game and settle in for some pizza. The throbbing pain emanating from your ankle is distracting, and you continue to worry about what the immediate future holds. As you integrate into your home with your family, the afternoon's frustration releases into a degree of comfort and reassurance that your ankle will heal and you will return to normal, everyday functions at some point.

You follow Dr. Smith's suggestions, keep your foot elevated and iced, and note the increased pain when the Advil wears off. You are restless all night due to the discomfort and anxiety. The new day brings an array of pinks, blues, and yellows to your leg, in addition to the swelling. You guess the colors are normal but note the added element of anxiety, as the rainbow was an unexpected and surprising sight. You still don't know if you have a broken bone. Wearing your soft ankle brace, you make it to work, thanks to help from your kids and your spouse.

EXHIBIT 3-3 CARE INDEX

	INTERACTION WITH PATIENT	EFFECT ON STRESS/FEAR	CARE RATING
DR. SMITH'S RECEPTIONIST	Disorganized, unfriendly, and distracted; added to stress; wasted time	Unnecessary annoyance	Poor
APPARENT NURSE (SALLY)	Cold, mechanical, hurried, possibly unqualified	Added fear and stress by saying, "It could get worse if you walk on it," and offering no solution or comfort	Fair
DR. SMITH	Little to no interest in the patient's life or stress level	Added stress by indicating that it might be broken; increased fear with no outlet to diffuse the fear because of indifference to personal circumstances	Fair
RADIOLOGIST RECEPTIONIST	Rude, disrespectful, unhelpful	Added stress; increased frustration; no effect on fear	Poor
X-RAY TECH-NOLOGIST	Friendly, caring, forthright, honest, qualified	Reduced stress; reassuring	Excellent

Luckily, you have a desk job, and you can prop your foot up for most of the day while performing your work. As the afternoon wears on, your ability to focus on work diminishes as you await the call from Dr. Smith's office. Lunchtime gives way to afternoon, and you can no longer stand the wait. You think, "It's been twenty-four hours and Denise said Dr. Smith's office would have the report in twenty-four hours." You call Dr. Smith's office. It's 4:45.

You are greeted with, "Dr. Smith's office, hold please." Three more minutes added to your lifetime lost. You wait on hold, and finally the receptionist picks up and says, "How can I help you?" You state your name and that you are waiting for results of your X-ray.

The receptionist states, "When we get the reports, we will call you." You indicate that you are in discomfort and would really like your results. She says, "Hold, please."

EXHIBIT 3-4 ANXIETY LEVEL FOLLOWING RADIOLOGY

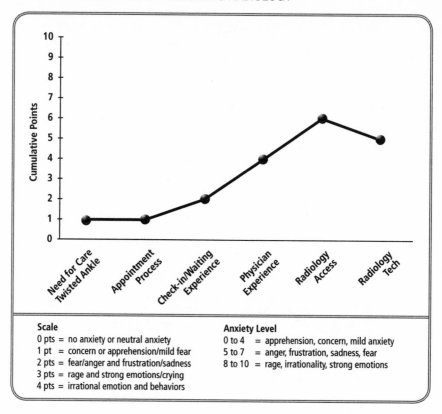

Scale
0 pts = no anxiety or neutral anxiety
1 pt = concern or apprehension/mild fear
2 pts = fear/anger and frustration/sadness
3 pts = rage and strong emotions/crying
4 pts = irrational emotion and behaviors

Anxiety Level
0 to 4 = apprehension, concern, mild anxiety
5 to 7 = anger, frustration, sadness, fear
8 to 10 = rage, irrationality, strong emotions

The hold time is upward of five to seven minutes. Finally, the line is picked up and a person hastily says, "This' Sally."

You restate your name and the request for the results from the X-ray taken yesterday. Sally states, "We will call you when we get the report."

You indicate you are in discomfort and were hoping to learn about your X-ray. Sally says, "Hold on."

Ten minutes later, the receptionist picks up the phone, and asks, "Who are you waiting for?" You restate your name and indicate you are waiting for Sally, who is getting your results. The receptionist says, "Okay, hold on."

Sally picks up the line and indicates she does not have your results. You say, "Denise at the radiology office said Dr. Smith would have the results in twenty-four hours."

Sally says, "We don't have it; who is Denise?"

You respond, "Denise is the person who took the X-ray. What should we do?"

"She shouldn't have told you we would have the report in twenty-four hours. We never get them that fast unless it's a stat."

With mounting frustration, you ask why your X-ray wasn't a stat. Sally responds, "Your injury certainly wasn't life threatening, and you weren't in excruciating pain; it's not a stat situation."

"Well," you ask, "when *can* I expect my results?" Silently, you are wondering how many life-threatening situations would survive the receptionist's hold time.

Sally says, "We should have them tomorrow." It's 5:05.

Case Analysis

LOST LIFETIME

Lost lifetime: 20 minutes
Cumulative lost lifetime: 127 minutes (2 hours 7 minutes)

To this point, the patient has lost more than two hours of her life to the inefficient access and uncaring communication, with no sign of resolution on the horizon.

CARE INDEX

Exhibit 3-5 charts the level of care provided by the doctor's receptionist and nurse.

ANXIETY LEVEL

Exhibit 3-6 shows the graph of anxiety levels, adding in family time, which reduced anxiety, and the wait for test results.

For the second consecutive day you arrive home frustrated and in pain. The fear your ankle is broken is mounting. What if you need surgery? What if it takes three months to heal? How will you continue with your life's activities? How will you have fun? Your anger invokes the desire to kick something, but you also realize kicking may not be the most prudent choice to vent your frustration. Tears begin to flow. How come your X-ray wasn't a stat? How come they didn't even tell you *stat* existed? Why are they all so rude? Don't they know you expect them to care for you?

As your mind wanders, you cling to the thought that you certainly won't die because of this injury but your lifestyle has been compromised, not only by the injury but also by the lack of communication and care received from your alleged caregivers. Why isn't the report available when they said it would be? You and Denise agreed that Dr. Smith would have it in twenty-four hours. When will someone help you? When will someone care about you? You resolve that you will call Denise first thing in the morning.

You call the radiologist's office at 8:30 the next morning. The receptionist answers, you state your name and that your radiology report was supposed to be faxed to Dr. Smith's office yesterday but they didn't get it.

The receptionist asks, "When did you have your exam?"

You respond, "The day before yesterday."

The receptionist states, "All of our reports are faxed no later than twenty-four hours from the exam, except for mammograms. You didn't have a mammogram, did you?"

"No, I had an X-ray of my ankle."

The receptionist responds, "Then your report was faxed yesterday."

You indicate, "No, Dr. Smith's office didn't have it when I spoke with them late yesterday."

The debate continues as the receptionist responds, "They have it; they just haven't filed it yet."

You ask, "Can I speak with Denise?"

The receptionist questions, "The tech? She is seeing patients; you can't talk to her."

With frustration seeping into your tone you request, "Can she return a call to me?"

EXHIBIT 3-5 CARE INDEX

	INTERACTION WITH PATIENT	EFFECT ON STRESS/FEAR	CARE RATING
DR. SMITH'S RECEPTIONIST	Disorganized, unfriendly, and distracted; added to stress; wasted time	Unnecessary annoyance	Poor
APPARENT NURSE (SALLY)	Cold, mechanical, hurried, possibly unqualified	Added fear and stress by saying, "It could get worse if you walk on it," and offering no solution or comfort	Fair
DR. SMITH	Little to no interest in the patient's life or stress level	Added stress by indicating that it might be broken; increased fear with no outlet to diffuse the fear because of indifference to personal circumstances	Fair
RADIOLOGIST RECEPTIONIST	Rude, disrespectful, unhelpful	Added stress; increased frustration; no effect on fear	Poor
X-RAY TECH-NOLOGIST	Friendly, caring, forth-right, honest, qualified	Reduced stress; reas-suring	Excellent
DR. SMITH'S RECEPTIONIST	Rude, disrespectful, unhelpful, unfriendly, distracted	Added stress; neutral effect on fear	Poor
APPARENT NURSE (SALLY)	Cold, mechanical, sys-tematic, unprofessional (scapegoating Denise at the radiologist's office), not resolution oriented	Added stress; neutral effect on fear	Poor

Your response is met with, "I will give her a message, but I don't know when she will get back to you."

Your frustration is rapidly transitioning to anger. "If she doesn't call by two, I am going to call you back."

The receptionist repeats, "I don't know when she can call you, and I don't know if she will call you by two."

EXHIBIT 3-6 ANXIETY LEVEL: WAITING GAME

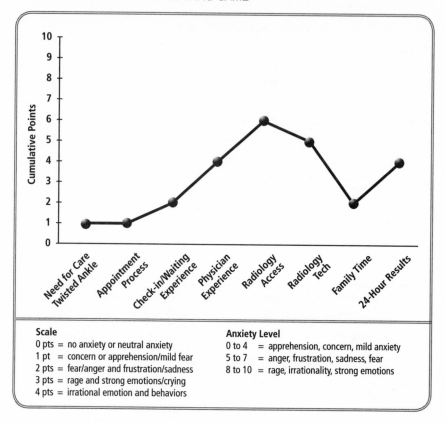

Scale
0 pts = no anxiety or neutral anxiety
1 pt = concern or apprehension/mild fear
2 pts = fear/anger and frustration/sadness
3 pts = rage and strong emotions/crying
4 pts = irrational emotion and behaviors

Anxiety Level
0 to 4 = apprehension, concern, mild anxiety
5 to 7 = anger, frustration, sadness, fear
8 to 10 = rage, irrationality, strong emotions

You ask, "What is your name?" The receptionist says her name is Dawn. Suppressing the rising anger in your tone, you say, "Dawn, I trust you will give my message to Denise when we hang up."

She responds, "I can't leave my desk. I can only give it to her when she comes to the waiting room to get a patient."

It's 8:38.

You call Dr. Smith's office, navigate your way to Sally's line, only to get her voice mail. You leave her a message to call you ASAP, as the radiologist's receptionist claims her office sent the report yesterday.

It's 8:52.

At 10:48, Denise returns your call. She validates that the report was faxed to Dr. Smith yesterday at 1:47 p.m. per the fax log listed in her computer system. You call Dr. Smith's office again and demand to speak with

Sally. After a combined hold time of eight minutes, Sally picks up the line, "This' Sally."

You state your name and ask her why she hadn't returned your call from earlier. She says that she returns all messages at 11:30 each day. (Your thought: "It would be nice if her voice mail said that.")

You indicate that Denise at the radiologist's office claims your report was faxed yesterday at 1:47 p.m. You ask Sally to look for the results.

She sighs and says, "It's probably on his desk."

"Well, go find it on his desk, and call me back before 11:30."

Sally responds, "I'll try, but I can't guarantee he will read it by then."

Until this moment, the thought that Dr. Smith hadn't read your report hadn't crossed your mind. Surely Dr. Smith cares enough about you that he has read the report by now! As your mind wanders to acts of desperate behavior to get Dr. Smith's attention, you request to speak with Dr. Smith directly.

Sally says, "Why do you need to speak with Dr. Smith?"

You respond, "Because, I need to ask him to read my report and tell me what I need to do."

Sally says, "I can leave him a message to call you, but he won't call you before 4:45."

You ask, "Will he have read my report by then?"

"He usually gets to them, but we are really busy today, I would hope that by 4:45 he would have read it, but I can't guarantee that."

You confirm with Sally that she is going to call you at 11:30 whether she has the report or not. She responds, "I'll try."

As you hang up the phone, you suppress tears of frustration and bang your fist on your desk in anger. It's 11:10.

Case Analysis

LOST LIFETIME

Lost lifetime: 22 minutes
Cumulative lost lifetime: 149 minutes (2 hours 29 minutes)

CARE INDEX

Exhibit 3-7 charts the care provided by the receptionist and nurse on this occasion.

ANXIETY LEVEL

Exhibit 3-8 charts the anxiety level to this point.

Finally, Results

No surprise—11:30 comes and goes, and you don't hear from Sally. A co-worker invites you to lunch, and the pleasant diversion is welcomed. There is a voice mail when you return. It's Michelle from Dr. Smith's office calling on his behalf. She would like you to return her call. You think to yourself, "Who the heck is Michelle?"

You promptly call Michelle, wade through the receptionist's pleasures, and disappointingly reach Michelle's voice mail. You leave a very clear and assertive message for Michelle, stating you are in significant discomfort and need a return call ASAP. You also call the receptionists at your work place and put them on alert for any calls for you from Dr. Smith's office. It is 11:45.

At 2:10, Michelle returns your call. She is a seemingly upbeat, happy person who indicates she is calling on behalf of Dr. Smith to let you know your X-ray is normal. You take the opportunity to breathe a sigh of relief and proceed to ask Michelle what your next steps toward healing should be.

The overwhelming feeling of relief supersedes your normal thought process, and you forget to ask Michelle for her credentials or experience level. She indicates you should continue to keep your foot elevated, walk as little as possible, use ice and Advil as needed, and check in with Dr. Smith next Wednesday.

EXHIBIT 3-7 CARE INDEX: TRYING TO GET RESULTS

	INTERACTION WITH PATIENT	EFFECT ON STRESS/FEAR	CARE RATING
RADIOLOGIST RECEPTIONIST	Rude, disrespectful, unhelpful	Added stress; increased frustration; no effect on fear	Poor
X-RAY TECH-NOLOGIST	Friendly, caring, forth-right, honest, qualified	Reduced stress; reassuring	Excellent
DR. SMITH'S RECEPTIONIST	Unfriendly, distracted, inefficient	Added stress because of inefficiencies	Poor
APPARENT NURSE (SALLY)	Cold, mechanical, hurried, possibly unqualified	Barrier to wellness and stress reduction; added fear and frustration because of noncommittal responses	Poor
DR. SMITH	Inaccessible	Added stress because of unavailability of care provider	Poor
DR. SMITH'S RECEPTIONIST	Rude, disrespectful, unhelpful, unfriendly, distracted	Added stress; neutral effect on fear	Poor
APPARENT NURSE (SALLY)	Cold, mechanical, sys-tematic, unprofessional (scapegoating Denise at the radiologist's office), not resolution oriented	Added stress; neutral effect on fear	Poor

Before you let Michelle go, you ask, "When did Dr. Smith receive my report from the radiologist?"

There is a moment of swooshing paper and she responds, "It came in yesterday afternoon."

It's 2:20.

Michelle transfers you to the receptionist to schedule your follow-up appointment. You hear, "Dr. Smith's office, hold please." The cycle begins again.

EXHIBIT 3-8 ANXIETY LEVEL: PHONE TAG

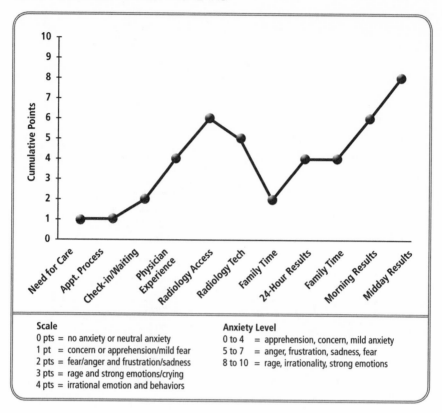

Scale
0 pts = no anxiety or neutral anxiety
1 pt = concern or apprehension/mild fear
2 pts = fear/anger and frustration/sadness
3 pts = rage and strong emotions/crying
4 pts = irrational emotion and behaviors

Anxiety Level
0 to 4 = apprehension, concern, mild anxiety
5 to 7 = anger, frustration, sadness, fear
8 to 10 = rage, irrationality, strong emotions

Final Case Analysis

LOST LIFETIME

Lost lifetime: 15 minutes
Cumulative lost lifetime: 164 minutes (2 hours 44 minutes)

ANXIETY LEVEL

Exhibit 3-9 shows the final anxiety chart for this scenario, from the point of injury until the good news was delivered.

What Should Have Happened

At this stage, does it really matter who made the mistake, Dr. Smith or the radiologist's office? No. This patient experienced a direct loss of nearly three hours of her life due to an ineffective access system, and she isn't done yet. She has to go back in a week and experience the same inefficiencies.

In addition to the systematic inefficiencies, note how this patient began her health care experience. She was excited about her life. Her son's Little League team just won the tournament. By the end of the encounter she was angry, stressed, disappointed, and then finally relieved to hear the bone was not broken. The injury to her ankle was enough of a life disruption without her doctor adding fear of the unknown ("It might be broken,") and without most staff members contributing rudeness, disrespect, and incompetence.

A Better Way

Regretfully many of us are too familiar with this sort of encounter. What if the previous encounter could function like this?

You call your doctor's office and hear, "Dr. Smith's office; this is Tom. How can I care for you?" You state you have twisted your ankle at your son's Little League game and need an appointment.

Tom replies, "The first available time is 2:30; will you be okay for two hours?"

You respond, "Yes, I can get through the next two hours. I have taken some Advil, but it's really swollen."

Tom says, "Okay, we will see you at 2:30. Did they win?" His question brings a smile to your face and you respond with a resounding yes!

You arrive for your appointment at 2:26 p.m. and are greeted by Mike, the receptionist. When he sees you open the door limping, he meets you at the door and offers you his arm, saying, "My name is Mike, have a seat." Mike requests your driver's license and insurance card and takes them to his computer. Mike returns to you and says, "Your co-payment for today's

EXHIBIT 3-9 ANXIETY LEVEL: FINAL RESULTS

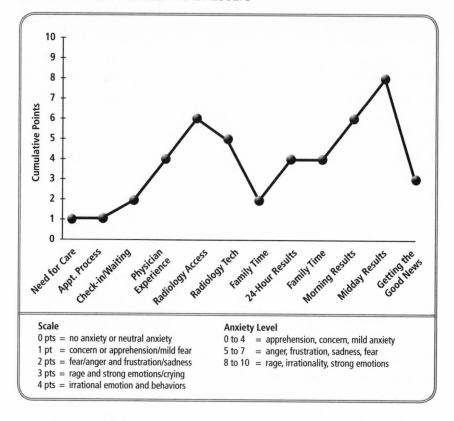

Scale
0 pts = no anxiety or neutral anxiety
1 pt = concern or apprehension/mild fear
2 pts = fear/anger and frustration/sadness
3 pts = rage and strong emotions/crying
4 pts = irrational emotion and behaviors

Anxiety Level
0 to 4 = apprehension, concern, mild anxiety
5 to 7 = anger, frustration, sadness, fear
8 to 10 = rage, irrationality, strong emotions

visit is twenty-five dollars." You give him your debit card and he takes care of the charge. It's now 2:32.

At 2:33, Sally, Dr. Smith's nurse, enters the reception area. When your eyes meet, a big smile comes to her face as she greets you and offers you her arm. As you limp to the exam room, Sally says, "Now I understand the Little League game got you excited, you've got considerable swelling in your ankle, and you've taken some Advil to get you through the last two hours. Is there anything new you need to add?"

You respond, "We were at Danny's Little League game, he plays short-stop. It was the last inning of the tournament game and they were winning by one run. Bases were loaded and the other team's heavy hitter was at bat.

It was spine tingling; all the parents were on the edge of their seats. The batter hit a hard ground ball practically into left field, Danny grabbed it, tagged the runner going to third out, threw the ball to first, got the batter out, game over. We won! In all the winning excitement, I was jumping up and down on the bleachers and twisted my ankle."

Sally, still offering that warming smile, responds, "Danny is how old now, eight?" As Sally takes your vital signs, Dr. Smith enters the exam room. It's 2:43.

He walks up to you with a grin. "I heard they won." You respond with a smile and a resounding "Yes they did." Your ankle is throbbing badly and the pain is beginning to take over your entire being. Dr. Smith says, "Well, let's look at this ankle and see what we can do to get you back on track." As he examines your ankle, your mind wanders to all the things you need to get done.

Dr. Smith says, "I would like for you to get your ankle X-rayed, just to be certain nothing is broken." Sally is going to get you a brace to help support your ankle while you walk, and you should keep taking the Advil for inflammation. How does that sound?"

You respond, "That sounds fine. Do you really think it's broken?"

Dr. Smith's face illuminates into a warm smile, and he places a comforting hand on your shoulder. He looks you in the eye and says, "Even if it is broken, it will heal, and you will be fine." Dr. Smith leaves the exam room.

Sally returns with written instructions to use ice and Advil, reminds you to keep your foot elevated above your heart, and gives you the soft brace for you to wear until the results of the X-ray are returned. It's 2:57.

Feeling sad and frustrated, you hold Sally's arm and limp back to Mike in the receptionist area. You wonder how you are going to get dinner together. Mike greets you with a smile and indicates that Dr. Smith will call you tomorrow between 1:00 and 2:00 with your X-ray results. He offers you his arm or a wheelchair to head down to suite 101, where the X-ray office is located. You choose his arm. It's 3:05 when you arrive in the radiologist's office.

Case Analysis: A Better Way

LOST LIFETIME

The care associated with this encounter wastes none of your time.

Appointment start time:	2:30
Completion time:	3:05
Total time:	35 minutes
	-30 minutes with Dr. Smith and Sally
	- 5 minutes (personal expectation for clerical interactions)
Lost lifetime:	0 minutes
Cumulative lost lifetime:	0 minutes

CARE INDEX

No need for a detailed chart here; the care can be summarized in one word: positive.

- Receptionists Mike and Tom: caring helpful, positive, competent
- Sally: caring, concerned, qualified
- Dr. Smith: caring, positive, respectful
- Fear: decreasing
- Anxiety/frustration: neutral
- Care rating: excellent
- Ancillary care rating: excellent

ANXIETY LEVEL

Exhibit 3-10 shows the chart for this ideal scenario.

BACK TO THE RADIOLOGIST

When you and Mike enter the radiologist's office, the waiting area is about half-filled with other patients. You are greeted by Stephanie, the receptionist. Tom has faxed all of your data to her, and she is expecting you. She indicates the wait will be approximately ten minutes. It's 3:12. You take a seat.

At 3:18 an X-ray technologist snuggles a wheelchair up next to where you are sitting. "My name is Denise; I am a registered X-ray technologist. I heard your son's team won today. Now, what is going on with that ankle?"

You respond, "I twisted my ankle at my son's Little League game, and it really hurts."

"That's too bad; I can see you are in pain. Your son plays what position?"

You respond, "He plays shortstop. Do you think my ankle is broken?"

Denise says she doesn't know if your ankle is broken, but that she will be sure to take a clear picture for the radiologist so she can see for certain what is going on. Denise proceeds to take three pictures of your ankle. As Denise sends you home, she indicates the results of your X-ray will be faxed to Dr. Smith's office and Dr. Smith will call you tomorrow between 1:00 and 2:00 p.m. with the results.

You ask Denise if the results can be sent to you directly and as soon as they are ready. Denise indicates that she can send you the results as well, but warns you not to be frustrated if some of the medical terminology is challenging to understand. You provide her with your fax number.

Somewhat deflated by the impending twenty-four-hour wait to find out if your ankle is broken, you thank Denise for her care. Denise asks you if you need a cab or would like wheelchair assistance to your car. You feel able to drive, but would welcome a ride to your car. Its 3:45; you are on your way to pick up Sandy at soccer practice and head home.

EXHIBIT 3-10 ANXIETY LEVEL: THE BETTER WAY

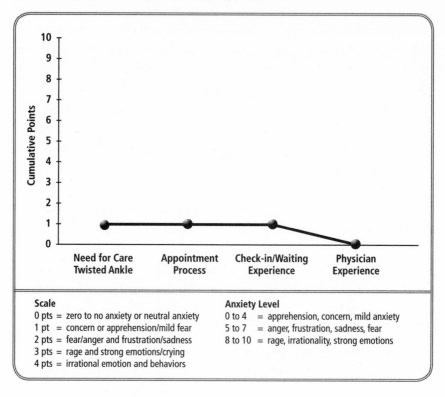

Case Analysis

LOST LIFETIME

Appointment start time:	3:12
Completion time:	3:45
Total time	33 minutes
	-21 minutes with Denise
	- 5 minutes (personal expectation for clerical interactions)
Lost lifetime:	7 minutes
Cumulative lost lifetime:	7 minutes

CARE INDEX

- Receptionist: friendly, competent, efficient, no repeated steps, and connected to the other receptionist
- Radiology technologist: friendly, caring, forthright, honest, qualified, reassuring
- Fear: decreasing
- Anxiety/frustration: decreasing
- Care rating: excellent (personal expectation standards)
- Ancillary care rating: excellent

ANXIETY LEVEL

Exhibit 3-11 rates the anxiety level of the patient under this new, improved scenario.

Your family welcomes your arrival home. Again, you congratulate Danny for a great game and settle in for some pizza. The throbbing pain emanating from your ankle is distracting, and you continue to worry about what the immediate future holds. As you integrate into your home with your family, the afternoon's frustration releases into a degree of comfort and reassurance that your ankle will heal and you will return to normal functions at some point.

You follow Dr. Smith's suggestions and keep your foot elevated and iced, noting the increased pain when the Advil wears off. The night is laden with restlessness, as you don't sleep well due to the pain and anxiety of your injury. The new day brings an array of pinks, blues, and yellows, in addition to the swelling, just as Sally said might occur. Her note indicated the colors are a sign of the normal healing process, and not to worry about them. Wearing your soft ankle brace, you make it to work, thanks to the help from your kids and your spouse.

EXHIBIT 3-11 IDEAL ANXIETY LEVEL

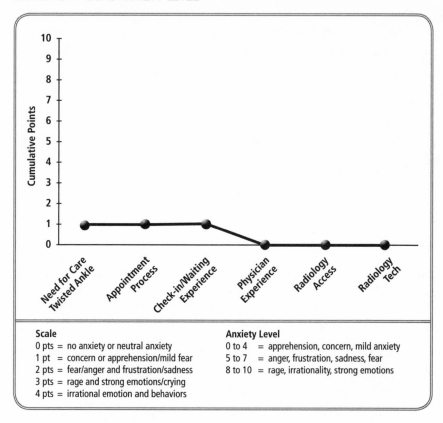

Scale		Anxiety Level	
0 pts	= no anxiety or neutral anxiety	0 to 4	= apprehension, concern, mild anxiety
1 pt	= concern or apprehension/mild fear	5 to 7	= anger, frustration, sadness, fear
2 pts	= fear/anger and frustration/sadness	8 to 10	= rage, irrationality, strong emotions
3 pts	= rage and strong emotions/crying		
4 pts	= irrational emotion and behaviors		

Luckily, your job is a desk job, and you can prop your foot up for most of the day. When you return from lunch, a fax from the radiologist is awaiting your arrival. Some of the jargon is foreign to you, but the clear message is there are no broken bones. At 1:30, Dr. Smith calls with an affirmation of the good news: no breaks. He provides you with a care plan that seems reasonable and will work with your life. He passes the call to Mike so you can book a follow-up appointment.

When Mike picks up the line he says, "Laura?" to which you respond "yes." He continues, "I am so glad your ankle isn't broken." You and he then proceed to find a mutually agreed upon date for your next visit.

Mike ends the call with "You know you can call for Sue anytime, and she can answer your questions or concerns, right? If you have concerns after we have gone for the day, you can call and have us paged. If you have a computer at home, you can page us via e-mail or utilize our nurses' online service. This service can access your chart notes with your permission, and then you can enter into a live chat with a nurse. All of the nurses are experienced, qualified RNs, or registered nurses. They will log your conversation in your chart and we will check in with you in the morning." Mike gives you Dr. Smith's online ID number in case you want to utilize the chat service.

Final Case Analysis

LOST LIFETIME

Lost lifetime: 0 minutes
Cumulative lost lifetime: 7 minutes

CARE INDEX

- Receptionists: friendly, caring, and competent
- Radiology office: competent
- Dr. Smith: competent, caring, and professional
- Fear: none
- Anxiety/frustration: decreasing
- Care rating: excellent
- Ancillary care rating: excellent

ANXIETY LEVEL: FINAL ANALYSIS

The revised version of this experience diminishes anger and frustration, thus allowing the patient to focus primarily on healing. The results are presented in exhibit 3-12.

EXHIBIT 3-12 ANXIETY LEVEL: FINAL ANALYSIS

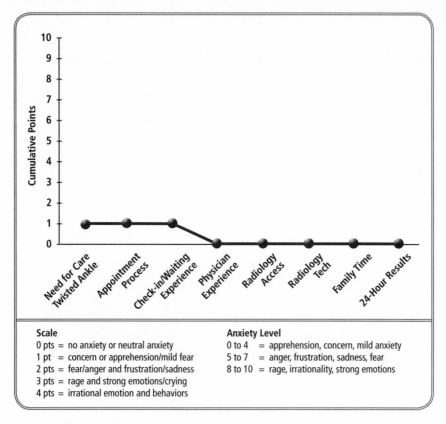

Scale
0 pts = no anxiety or neutral anxiety
1 pt = concern or apprehension/mild fear
2 pts = fear/anger and frustration/sadness
3 pts = rage and strong emotions/crying
4 pts = irrational emotion and behaviors

Anxiety Level
0 to 4 = apprehension, concern, mild anxiety
5 to 7 = anger, frustration, sadness, fear
8 to 10 = rage, irrationality, strong emotions

How to Navigate When It's Your Ankle

Let's review this encounter one last time with the addition of speaking points and options to assist you when you encounter a challenging access system. The speaking points have been added to assist you with words and confidence when you encounter an unfriendly or inefficient access system. The original scenario is in italics, followed by the speaking points.

You call your doctor's office and hear, "Dr. Smith's office, please hold." If this is a new provider you have never seen before, one option is to hang up and call another office. If you want to assess whether this greeting is the norm, you could call back in thirty minutes and see if you receive the same "hold please" greeting and then make a decision as to whether to move on to a different provider or persevere with this one. When you finally speak with the receptionist, you say, "My name is Laura Casey. What is your name?" Note the name of the receptionist in your personal medical record file. Then say, "Dawn, I value my time, and you just kept me on hold for three minutes. I twisted my ankle at my son's Little League game and need an appointment. I expect to be seen today, and I expect to wait no more than ten minutes past my designated appointment time before I am interacting with Dr. Smith."

If the access system is poor, Dawn won't be able to accommodate this request. If Dawn cannot make that commitment, you could request to speak with the office manager.

If you do speak with the manager, start over. "My name is Laura Casey. What is your name?" Note the name of the office manager in your personal medical record file. Then say, "David, I value my time. Are you aware that just about every time I call here I am placed on hold for one to three minutes? At this point, my interaction with you and your staff has just kept me on hold for six minutes, and I haven't yet accomplished my goal to book an appointment. I twisted my ankle at my son's Little League game and need an appointment. I expect to be seen today, and I expect to wait no more than ten minutes past my designated appointment time before I am interacting with Dr. Smith."

David may not be willing to make the commitment either. It's your choice as to how far up the management chain you would like to go to get a commitment. Minimally, you have made both David and Dawn aware of your expectations, and if they care, they will do their best to get Dr. Smith to you in a timely fashion.

Let's Continue

She indicates she can squeeze you in at 2:30 that afternoon. You arrive for your appointment at 2:26 and are greeted by a receptionist who is on the phone and sequestered behind a glass window. She isn't smiling and doesn't introduce herself. She hands you a clipboard of paperwork and a pen, and points to another clipboard. "Sign in," she says, phone still pressed to her ear, "and I will need a copy of your insurance card."

Don't comply with any of the requests. Wait for the receptionist to get off the phone and make her make eye contact with you. Simply stand there until she is done with her call. She will most likely repeat her request while she is on the line; just wait.

Once she is off the phone, say, "Are you Dawn? Dawn, it's a pleasure to meet you. Offer to shake her hand and introduce yourself. My name is Laura Casey, I am here for my 2:30 appointment with Dr. Smith. I can't sign your log because it's open for public view and that is not compliant with privacy law. However, here is my insurance card and my debit card for my $25 co-pay. I did want to remind you that I expect to be interacting with Dr. Smith by 2:40 at the latest."

If Dawn's response is anything but, "Absolutely, Ms. Casey," I suggest you simply ignore Dawn's response, as you have had the opportunity to state your expectations and Dawn is completely ill-equipped to even acknowledge those expectations. The point is you *communicated* them. Engaging with the likes of Dawn will only add to your stress level. Know your audience and choose with whom you are going to vent your frustration. Venting to Dawn will be ineffective. Providing constructive criticism to the CEO or physician is a better use of your time.

Find a seat close to the reception desk and continue to track your experience on your personal medical record.

Even though you have stated your expectations clearly, understand Dr. Smith's staff may not be able to meet your expectations. Therefore, you need to maintain your personal walk-out time. By walk-out time, I mean how long you will wait before you will actually walk out the door without receiving care. Know your boundary, communicate it, and stick to it. Please understand I am not advocating that you forgo care of a critical nature. If your health status is critical and you need care immediately, then receive the care you need, but note the service level as acceptable or unacceptable for future reference.

At 2:40, you have a couple options. You can get up and limp to the receptionist's desk, or you can attempt to get Dawn's attention from your seat (or ask another patient who is able to walk to request that Dawn come to you). If Dawn attempts to converse with you from the reception window, say, "Dawn, shouting across the waiting area doesn't comply with privacy law. It hurts for me to walk, so could you please come where I am so we can have a modicum of privacy?"

Expect an annoyed Dawn to arrive at your side. Smile and say, "Thank you for coming over here. It is 2:40, and I will wait another X minutes before leaving, at which point I will find another doctor for me and my family. Can you please convey that to David, the office manager? Also Dawn, if I intend to leave at X o'clock, I expect that you will come get my debit card at that time and credit my co-pay to my account."

If she wants your debit card now, don't give it to her. Make her come back to you at the designated time. The other goal is to point out they are losing not only your health care dollars but your *entire* family's health care dollars. Dawn won't understand that, but David should.

Use that good ol' American consumer power to divert your health care dollars to a provider who better suits your access needs and expectations. Hopefully you don't have to leave and find other care, but it's vitally important that you honor your words and do exactly what you outlined. If you do leave, write a letter to the doctor and copy David, the office manager, outlining why you and your entire family's care has been redirected to Dr. Jones's office. Let them know all the wonderful things about Dr. Jones's office and why you believe it to be a more suitable environment.

A person who appears to be a nurse calls your name out to the entire waiting room, and you hobble to the exam room. No, you don't. Motion to the nurse to come to where you are sitting. Say, "My name is Laura. What is yours?" Sally, I have injured my ankle, can you please offer me your arm?" As you walk with Sally say, "Sally, are you a registered nurse?"

If Sally is not a registered nurse and you are interested in her level of training, ask her how many years she attended school to reach her current level. Then ask how long she has worked as a licensed practice nurse or LPN? Chapter 4 provides definitions for clinician credentials.

When you finally get to Dr. Smith, recap your entire experience to the moment before the exam begins. Be sure to include how much of your lifetime has been lost and discuss whether you will stay with his practice if this level of service continues. Once you've said your piece, then commence with the exam.

. . . You react, "Broken?" It can't be broken! I have to take the Cub Scouts camping this weekend, I promised to help the coach get Danny's team ready for the next tournament game, and of course, I need to work tomorrow. You realize Danny's team won today, don't you? They are going to the state championship!"

Politely indifferent, Dr. Smith smiles and congratulates you on behalf of Danny. He hands you a referral form to get your ankle X-rayed and says he will be back in touch when he gets a report from the radiologist. Sally will be back to tell you what to do in the meantime. You need to communicate that the thought of a broken ankle has just raised your stress level higher than it was two seconds ago. Ask him to wait until you compose yourself, and then ask all the questions you can muster: Should I walk on it? How long will the X-ray take? When will I know if it's broken? If it's broken will I need a cast? Surgery? What if I have more questions later? How do I reach you? Since the doctor just caused your anxiety level to rise, it's important that he answer your questions and quell your apprehension.

Write down the answers! Don't allow him to leave until you have asked all of your questions, are satisfied with the answers, and have diminished the stress-level spike that the fear of a broken ankle provoked. If the doctor has left your exam room and you have more questions, ask the nurse to have him come back.

LET'S CONTINUE

Before leaving Dr. Smith's office, ask for copies of your personal and insurance information. Bring these copies to the radiology office.

. . . As you hobble to the radiologist's office you call your spouse and make arrangements for Sandy to get picked up from soccer practice, and you suggest pizza for the kids for dinner; you don't know when you will get home. You enter the radiologist's office. The waiting area is about half-filled with other patients. It's 4:07.

You present your insurance card and the form from Dr. Smith's receptionist to the radiology receptionist. Present your insurance card to the radiology receptionist, along with the copies of your personal and insurance information you brought from the receptionist at Dr. Smith's office. Tell the radiology receptionist, "If you need more information from me I will be seated over here. It's painful for me to walk, so you will need to come over to where I am sitting. I believe I need authorization for X-rays. The number for you to call is on the copy of the insurance card. Can you please call and get the necessary authorization? If they need to speak with me, they can call my cell phone, or you can bring the phone over to me."

Participate—know enough about your insurance to communicate what the health care providers need to do for you, and make sure they do it.

... *Your ankle hurts, your ego hurts, you are sad and frustrated, you are missing the postgame celebration, and you have no idea what this woman is talking about.* You may be feeling emotional at this point, but hopefully the emotion is directly related to the injury and the fun you are missing. Hopefully, the stress pertaining to any ineptitude or incompetence you've encountered is diminished because you are in control of your *lifetime*; you are *participating* and *communicating*.

... *Your response is led with a little smile as you recall the winning play of the game. You describe the game to Denise as she takes three pictures of your ankle. As Denise sends you home, she indicates the results of your X-ray will be sent to Dr. Smith's office by this time tomorrow. You ask Denise if the results can be sent to you directly and as soon as they are ready. Denise indicates that she can send you the results, but that her office's policy is to send the results to your primary doctor first and then, if you want a copy after you converse with your doctor, she will be happy to send you a copy.* Ask Denise why you need to wait. Why can't she simply fax the information to your fax number? It's your body, your medical record, your life, and you want to actively participate in your care. If you expect your results within twenty-four hours, don't take no for answer. If Denise cannot commit to sending your results to you directly and quickly, then ask to speak with the office manager or clinic administrator. Give that person your fax number and phone number and say that as their patient, you expect to receive your results directly and within twenty-four hours.

... *You follow Dr. Smith's suggestions, keep your foot elevated and iced, and note the increased pain when the Advil wears off. You are restless all night due to the discomfort and anxiety. The new day brings an array of pinks, blues, and yellows to your leg, in addition to the swelling. You guess the colors are normal but note the added element of anxiety, as the rainbow was an unexpected and surprising sight. You still don't know if you have a broken bone.*

If your situation is not life threatening or urgent and if you have Internet access, the questions pertaining to your body's reaction could be researched online. There are a plethora of good consumer-oriented websites with sound information that may be able to answer your question and relieve some of the stress relating to your fear of the unknown. The American Board of Medical Specialties suggests www.mayoclinic.org as a credible site for answers to clinical questions.

Whether you have Internet access or not, most certainly call your physician and talk with the on-call doctor in an effort to diminish your stress if the Internet is not available or fruitful.

. . . With mounting frustration, you ask why your X-ray wasn't a stat. Sally responds, "Your injury certainly wasn't life threatening, and you weren't in excruciating pain; it's not a stat situation."

"Well," you ask, "when can I expect my results?" Silently, you are wondering how many life-threatening situations would survive the receptionist's hold time.

Sally's response is "We should have them tomorrow." It's 5:05.

If you don't have what you asked for from the radiologist's office by the mutually agreed upon time, call the person at the radiologist office who made the commitment and ask why you have not received your results. Request the person commit to the exact time he or she is going to fax your results to you, or if the results are not yet ready, request the person call you back in several hours with an update, and continue requesting updates until you have what you want.

Using These Tips to Get Better Service

Understand most of the requests made by the patient in the reworked case will be met with enormous resistance and possibly greater disrespect and rudeness than had the patient simply complied with the staff requests. I suggest you meet these situations head on with a smile and as much of a positive, polite demeanor as your illness will allow—and I suggest you pick your battles.

Despite the attitude or disrespect that might be spewed back at you when you ask a receptionist to use a copy of your personal information from your last visit, remain polite. Expect the requests be met with "I can't . . ." or "You have to . . ." or "We won't do that," and meet the resistance respectfully and assertively. If you sink to the level of the inept receptionist, your message will be lost, and you will most likely find yourself complying with the repetitive inefficient processes of the provider's system or finding a different provider.

Although the whole encounter may be frustrating and confrontational, stick to your personal goals and standards and communicate those expectations in a polite, steady tone, even when you believe the recipient deserves worse.

Remember as the customer, you have the power and you are in control of your care experience. If efficient access and superior ancillary service is a priority for you, then divert your health care dollars to a provider that has what you are looking for.

I earlier described the months of telling every single provider Mom and I encountered, "Mom is not herself, she is tired, forgetful, and nauseous all the time." Despite my mounting frustration I was levelheaded, professional, and respectful, until we met the doctor in the emergency room. Even with him, I didn't fly off the handle; there were no tears, no yelling, and no irrational rage. There was, however, intensity, focus, and persistence. I wouldn't take no for an answer at that stage. Quite often, the people with whom you are interacting thrive on the power they perceive to hold over you. Move on to someone who can understand you and can affect change for you (i.e., a manager, doctor, administrator, or CEO).

Remember the lab that wanted Mom to register in administration every week? I simply told the lab staff that we wouldn't be doing that. The staff responded with, "You have to." I responded, "No, we don't. You see, Mom doesn't have the time to spend on your repetitive tasks, she has grade IV brain cancer." At which point the lab worker called downstairs to the admitting office, while Mom's blood was drawn. It took about three instances of this exact encounter before they got it right. By week four, they would see us coming and know that they had to pick up the phone and do the admitting part.

Be prepared for the resistance. Essentially, you are asking for change. You are asking for things no one else has, or not many have, asked for in the past. Be prepared for some failures and make peace with the encounters that conclude unsuccessfully. In most cases you have treatment options and can make choices based on your personal expectations and the access system you encounter.

The question still remains, how come my car dealership has figured out how to provide me with superior, efficient customer service and access, while the health care industry, an industry whose focus is *care*, hasn't? More importantly, why do we, as consumers, put up with it?

Why do we put up with the poor service? Two theories seem to apply. We love the doctor and believe there is no one better to care for us, or we acquiesce to the cultural power structure inherent to our health-related encounters (meaning the caregiver will heal me), leaving our power behind. We put up with all kinds of inefficiencies and wrongs when we love the doctor or believe we are powerless to affect a change. Many patients leave their consumer power, thoughts, beliefs, and values at the door of the health care facility, and in doing so we perpetuate the mediocrity.

I began this book with the words "I am a person just like you." Your doctor is a person just like you, too. The fact that we bond with those who help us and help heal us is an extraordinarily important part of the healing process, but it does not absolve or shelter physicians and health care leaders from poor, unhealthy, disrespectful, and dysfunctional access systems.

If you love your doctor and would never seek care from someone else, but wade through the muck and lose precious moments of your lifetime every time you need his or her attention, then you need to start describing your losses to your doctor. In many cases, the physician is completely unaware of the reality associated with his or her access system. In some cases, the doctor may not care to know or participate in the enhancement of the access process. If the doctor doesn't care to be informed so that he or she can make improvements, you need to ask yourself, "Do I still love this doctor?"

There is no right or wrong answer to that question, and your answer may wax and wane with your health status. The question, however, is an important one to pose. If your lifetime is wasted because your doctor or the facility with which he or she is affiliated hasn't made good hiring choices, or hasn't figured out a friendly, efficient, competent access process, then that loss is a serious unrecoverable loss of your life. Be consciously aware of the choice you make when you continue your care with that doctor.

Remain focused on your personal goals. In general, the goal is to return to a status of health and wellness as efficiently and as stress free as possible. The first access example is not efficient. It adds stress to the patient's life because of poor communication and systematic inefficiencies that leave the consumer frustrated, fearful, and stressed.

Set your expectations pertaining to access and fire the poor performers. Long waits, rude staff, misinformation, and delayed information all sum to a disorganized access system that may be unacceptable to you. If you love the doctor, then figure out how to find the assertive voice to respectfully tell the doctor every time you see him or her what your access experience was like.

Confronting the doctor you love dearly with constructive criticism may not be the easiest conversation, but he or she needs to know the receptionist has no people skills and doesn't care about your personal well-being. There is stress relating to the confrontation and taking action. If you are going to remain a patient of this physician, then the way to enhance your access experiences is to communicate your desires and expectations clearly.

Allergic Reactions

When you don't have a relationship with the doctor, it's easier to fire the poor performer. Recently I went to see an allergist. I have had a known food allergy for about fifteen years, and a recent trip to the ER because my tongue was swelling prompted me to come out of denial and become a bit more focused on my situation. I searched for allergists on my insurance company's website. I chose an allergist based on the site's allergy classifications and called the provider.

Booking the appointment was simple and acceptable to me. During the appointment process there were no stipulations indicating I should arrive early to complete paperwork so I arrived at 3:01 for my 3:00 p.m. visit. The receptionist didn't smile, asked my name, requested a copy of my insurance card, and told me to sign in. I have a personal issue with sign-in sheets. They aren't confidential and they are the lazy way to attempt to keep the patients sitting in the waiting room in order of arrival. Each time I am required to sign one, I make my mark on the page and it's never legible. Then, I wait to see what they do when they can't read my name.

The nameless receptionist gave me forms to fill out, as this was my first visit. There was no pen on the clipboard. I asked to take the pen I used for the sign-in sheet. She approved, and I thought, well I guess the next person doesn't have to sign in.

I completed the forms and omitted my employer information. The sign-in sheet tipped me off that this practice doesn't quite understand all of the HIPAA privacy laws, and quite possibly will be inappropriate in other areas. (HIPAA is a law that requires health care providers to keep your health information private and only divulge it to necessary parties for very specific reasons and with your approval.) I wanted to see what Nameless would do with incomplete information. I gave her the clipboard and the pen. She returned my insurance card and asked me to sign another form three times.

The first signature was to acknowledge I have a co-payment, the second was to acknowledge my co-payment is due at the time of service, and the third said I would be billed $25 for missing appointments. "Wunderbar!" I thought sarcastically. "I am making a lot of commitments. I wonder what sort of commitments this practice is going to make on my behalf?"

I returned to my seat in the waiting room and sure enough, Nameless noted my missing employer information. She raised her voice to speak to me across the waiting room. She asked, "Laura do you have a work phone? You didn't fill this out, we need to be able to reach you at work." First I thought, "Why would my allergist have to reach me at work?"

Then I awkwardly answered, "Well, yes . . . I have a work phone . . . but don't call me there. Call my cell, 555-1234."

"What was the number?" she hollered across the waiting room. I repeated my cell phone number for everyone in the waiting room to hear.

As you might imagine, I was reacting to the extraordinary level of poor service associated with this initial encounter, and you may wonder why I gave the entire waiting room my cell phone number not once but twice. I did it because part of me wanted to see just how far the "wrong" would go, and the tone of my response made it clear to the entire waiting room the question and the whole interaction was completely inappropriate.

Requesting I shout my phone number across the waiting room set off alarms for me. "This person obviously had no couth, no concern for confidentiality, and no concept of the real world. Hasn't she seen the commercials on identity theft?" I thought. I guess she doesn't really care about much, and clearly not about me.

I settled into my book, and before I knew it, it was 3:20. I'd broken my own rule to not wait more than fifteen minutes to be seen. I was at a very interesting point in the book, so I read for another three minutes, packed up my book, and headed over to Nameless.

Please know I have walked out of many health care facilities due to poor service. I must share with you that I feel anxious as I make the commitment to leave and let the facility know why I am leaving. My heart rate goes up, and I have a definite physical reaction surrounding the impending confrontation. It's a hard thing to do. I think it's especially hard because we have been trained that doctors care for us. We understand doctors are meant to help us heal, and walking out on one creates anxiety for me. However, I believe walking out is my only option in this situation.

Nameless, who could double for Speechless at this stage, was at her computer terminal. When I approached the reception area she didn't acknowledge my presence. There happened to be a clinical staff member in the reception area as well. Awkwardly, I stood there for about thirty seconds. Despite the fact we were all within three feet of one another, neither of the women made eye contact or acknowledged my presence. I thought, maybe I had sprouted horns in the last twenty minutes, or possibly I had a large piece of mucus dangling from my nose and they didn't want to interact with me.

Finally, the clinical person broke the silence and asked if I had been helped. I said, "I need to reschedule." Nameless, who most certainly had transformed to Speechless, didn't move, didn't look up, and didn't speak. She continued typing. The clinical person and I made eye contact as we are waiting for Speechless to interact.

After another very pregnant pause, Speechless, still attentively focused on her computer screen, broke her silence and said, "Thursday at two or four."

WOW, reverberated through my head—she is truly an alien life form. I said, "I'll take your four." She maneuvered through the computer and gave me a reminder card. She uttered no other words.

Did I return to this provider? No way! I did call well in advance and cancel the appointment that I booked, and I most certainly chose to divert my health care dollars to a different provider. If it's okay for the reception-ist to communicate poorly, then why am I going to hang around to see what the provider's communication style is like? I decided to cut my losses and save my lifetime. Making this change was relatively easy because I had no emotional tie to the doctor, no bond needed to be broken, and I could simply redirect my dollars to another provider who would care for me.

A Different Waiting Room

I love the offices that believe your appointment began on time because they put you in an exam room on time. I liken this practice to the airlines logging a flight as departed on time because the plane was pushed back from the gate on time. They don't seem to count the time you spend sitting on the runway getting de-iced or waiting in line for other aircraft to take off.

Another group I recently fired for access issues was notorious for get-ting you in the exam room and leaving you there for thirty to forty min-utes (which, by the way, is a sign the doctor doesn't care). The purpose for my visit was to get a prescription refill. At the time of the appointment, I was quite healthy, so I certainly didn't leave any of my consumer power at the door and therefore would have no excuse to acquiesce to substandard service.

When I booked the appointment, my only requirement was to be the first patient of the day. I had an 8:00 a.m. appointment. I arrived at 7:55 and was greeted by the usual receptionist sequestered behind the glass panel who didn't introduce herself. I paid my co-payment and set up shop in the waiting area with my book.

At 8:02 the door to the waiting area opened and a woman in scrubs, in her best stage voice, called out, "Laura Casey." I gave her an A for timeliness, an F for confidentiality, and an internal eye roll, as I was the only person in the waiting room.

When we entered the exam room, she didn't tell me her name, she didn't tell me her credentials, and she didn't have any sort of ID badge or name tag. She took my blood pressure and pulse and told me I didn't have to sit up on the table—I could sit on the chair next to the desk. "Diane" would be right with me.

For the next seven or eight minutes, I read my book and blotted out the chatter outside the exam room door. At 8:10 I got up, left the exam room, and found the nameless woman in scrubs in the hall talking with another woman, who still had her jacket on and a purse slung over her shoulder. They were intently discussing someone's recent trip to Disney World. The nameless woman in scrubs was facing me and avoided eye contact with me. I would think she might be a bit concerned with the fact that at this stage I am the rogue patient AWOL from my exam room. I headed to the check-out station.

I got the receptionist's attention and asked how much longer the wait would be. The receptionist was a bit taken aback, as I was obviously on the wrong side of the window to be asking that question. She hesitantly responded, "You, you were in an exam room?" At this point, the nameless scrub woman rounded to corner, so I posed my question to her. As this interaction took place, the woman in the jacket with her purse scurried past us all.

The nameless scrub woman said, "She will be right with you."

I asked, "Is she with another patient?"

"No," responded the nameless scrub woman.

I added with a degree of intensity to my voice, "She isn't even *here* yet?"

The nameless scrub woman clarified, "No, she is here she is just . . . busy."

I said, "I see. Well, she has about two minutes to meet me in that room or I will be leaving."

I didn't really want to leave. The hassle associated with getting my co-pay back would most likely take an act of God for the receptionist to figure out. My goal was to escape as quickly as possible with my prescription. I returned to the exam room and purposefully left the door open.

By 8:15, the woman who had been wearing her jacket and had her purse slung over her shoulder entered my exam room. She didn't introduce herself, she didn't indicate what her credentials were. She sat down at the desk and, despite the tension in the room, asked me a couple questions about the prescription I needed and wrote the script.

As this was happening I began to waffle. I almost relinquished my consumer power to fear of confrontation. A little voice inside me said, "Wait a minute, this is wrong. I waited fifteen minutes so she could chit-chat with her buddy about Disney World?"

I said to the nameless clinician (presumably Diane), "You guys need to work on starting on time here in the mornings."

Her indignant response was, "It's customary to start at 8:15."

I concluded our meeting with, "Then your receptionist should tell me that so I am aware." The nameless apparent clinician had no response. As I left the office for the last time, I was glad I asked the timeliness question, because her response made it very clear that this practice not only has a broken access system, but the providers didn't care about my time, my opinion, or my life.

As I got in my car I remembered another telltale sign of missing care from this group. I recalled at the check-in counter a sign made out of bright pink, happy cardstock. Handwritten on the sign were the words, "Due to our new lease with ABC Health System, we no longer validate parking tickets for patients under 65."

First of all, what do I care about my provider's lease agreement with its building owner, and why is the provider laying blame on the landlord? Is that who I should be angry with about having to pay for my own parking? If my provider wanted to pay for my parking, then it could have cared enough to do that and made whatever other arrangements it needed to make with its landlord. Obviously, my provider cares enough for the Medicare patient population and is clearly inducing Medicare patients to obtain their care in an expense-free parking environment with disregard for non-Medicare patients.

On the surface the happy, pink, handmade sign is just tacky. Under scrutiny, the sign is all about money and scapegoating—not care. The message is a telltale sign pertaining to the values and focus of the management running the organization.

There *Are* Good Health Care Providers

On a positive note, I found a two-physician primary care practice that I need on occasion. Wendy, the receptionist, knows my name and has a basic understanding of my life. She asks about life and my work each time I see her. She tells me if my visit has been authorized by my insurance company. She is genuinely interested in me. When I do wait—and the wait has never exceeded my fifteen-minute limit—I watch Wendy interact with other patients. She is interested, respectful, and competent.

On one occasion I got trapped at work in an emotional meeting with one of my employees. I had to make the decision to be a no-show for my appointment, as it was inappropriate to end the discussion that was underway with my staff member. As soon as the meeting was over I phoned Wendy, because I felt awful for wasting the doctor's time. When she answered and learned it was me, her first question was, "Are you okay? It's not like you not to call if you can't make it." She understands me.

I explained what happened and apologized profusely. Wendy said, "No worries; the patient before you got here early. If you can come over now, we can put you in his slot." Do I love this woman? Absolutely. She understands, she is resolution-oriented, and she cares.

Generally, when you find yourself in a poor access system, communication is critical. Know your audience and hold the staff accountable to their commitments. If I book an appointment at 8:00 a.m., that means I expect to be visiting with the clinician at 8:00 a.m. If a staff member is privy to my personal information, I don't expect that staff member to leave it lying around for the next person to view. I don't expect the staff member to ask that I shout my phone number across the waiting room. I expect my access experience to be civilized, confidential, competent, caring, and anxiety-free.

Is waiting ever appropriate? Absolutely. I began this chapter with an analogy to an auto service department. My body certainly is not my automobile and there are nuances to health care delivery that are unlike any other industry. I used the auto service department analogy to help patients identify and understand what poor access systems look like. The decision to wait is the patient's choice and there are most certainly circumstances where waiting is warranted.

Health status will often drive your decision to wait longer than your personal standard. Most importantly, forgive the caring providers and facilities who have superior service when they are occasionally late to see you. Unlike the disorganized practice with poor communicators, the facility with excellent communication and care will be honest and explain their current situation. Generally they are going to be late because a patient walked through their door needing more care than everyone anticipated.

In this setting, staff will typically keep you apprised of how long the delay will be and with that information you can make your short-term choices. I'm not advocating you permanently leave a facility that provides superior care and service because they are late to see you one day. Caring providers are focused on delivering the appropriate level of care no matter how long it takes. Under these conditions, those of us in the waiting room should be thankful for the level of care available to all of us and especially to the person in need of the extra attention. Hopefully the day will never come when we need that level of service, but maintain peace of mind that you've found a good facility that cares and will attend to your needs.

Compass Points

Geography can create complex access situations. Living in one city and receiving care in another creates larger barriers to access and more communication breakdowns between patients, providers, and health systems. Mom's brain cancer was discovered in Chicago, her brain surgery took place in Chicago, but two weeks after her brain surgery, we needed her health care to flow on a continuum in Vermont.

Access is vitally important to the continuity of care. The complexities associated with distance and geography present a myriad of other challenges for patients. A friend travels two hours for his chemotherapy because he is part of a clinical trial. In addition to the burden and fear associated with his life-threatening illness and daily suffering, he and his wife must navigate access systems that say things like, "You aren't really our patient and therefore you have to . . ." Thus, they jump through all kinds of hoops, including redundant communication, just to keep everyone in sync.

How does a patient not really be someone's patient? Wouldn't we expect the system to care regardless of where one lives or where one's doctor lives? Communication systems break down across the miles. If you have a complex situation, expect to facilitate a lot of the communication between providers and their collective staff members. Expect to keep everyone on task and informed.

The nature of my friend's cancer is unique, and the disconnect between two health systems has educated them to be wary of communication across the miles. They need CT images taken on the same CT scanner each time staging is required. *Every* time the clinic schedules his CT exam they (the patient and his spouse) have to remind the health care delivery system who they are, that they must have a particular scanner, and that the reports and images need to be sent two hours down the highway. The systems are ill-equipped to manage the distance between the home community and the community where specialized care takes place. Faxes get lost, phone calls go unreturned, and quite often physician communication must be prodded along. All of this inefficiency is shouldered by the patient or his spouse, who acts as his advocate and supporter.

When you find yourself with a complicated access situation, I highly recommend you keep thorough documentation of all requests and commitments as discussed in chapter 5. Your heightened level of organization and communication will add precious moments to your lifetime.

Signs and Symptoms of a Poor Access System

When the people with whom you are working aren't doing what they said they were going to do, you need to pay close attention. Here are some other red flags.

- *Inflexibility* When staff members say, "We can't do that," or "I can't leave my work station to care for you," these are warning signals.

- *Scapegoating* "They never fax the report on time." "You have to pay to park because of the landlord."

- *Unfriendly behavior* Staff members who are rude, aloof, and make no eye contact or introductions.

- *Long waits*

- *Inefficient or redundant steps* "Your mom will have to go down to admissions and register for her blood work—*every* week."

- *Frequent staff turnover or physician turnover*

- *Lack of confidentiality* What can you hear about the care of others? What can you see relating to the care of others?

- *General disorganization of office functions*

Look for the stupidity. Calling out my name when I am the only person in the waiting room makes me wonder how present and attentive the person is going to be in the exam room. "Cute" handmade signs with ridiculous messages is another red flag. When you discover a poor access system, know you can divert your health care dollars if your health status permits.

Take you health care dollars elsewhere. Politely tell the provider why you are leaving, walk out, and find a provider who cares about and respects your time.

Write to the governing body of the health care organization and describe your experience. You'll need the following information:

- The practice administrator's name.
- The physician leader's name.
- The CEO's name.
- Where you should mail your correspondence.

If you choose to stay with the provider, then communicate to every person, including the provider, regarding the access and service levels. If your belief in that physician is correct, he or she will fix the problem and be grateful for your words.

Other tips to preserve your lifetime are

- Book your appointment via a manager or director in the organization.
- Document conversations.
- Outline your expectations (i.e., you won't wait more than X minutes to be interacting with the doctor).
- When access is complicated, plan to document the commitments of the people you encounter, and plan to communicate on their behalf and follow up with all parties to ensure that everyone is on the same page.

If you are stuck with a poor access system due to your insurance choices, take these steps:

1. Tell your HR department.
2. Change plans at next open enrollment period (if available).
3. Tell you health plan.

4. Formally complain to the State Department of Insurance, the Better Business Bureau, and the State Medical Society.

5. Set expectations and communicate those expectations effectively:

   - If my appointment is at 2:30, when can I expect to see the doctor?
   - Will a nurse see me prior to the doctor? Is the person a registered nurse?
   - How long shall I expect to be in your office from start to finish?
   - Why do you anticipate paperwork will take fifteen minutes?
   - Converse with other patients in the waiting room.
     - Is the wait always this long?
     - Is Dr. Smith really that good?
     - Is that nurse ever going to smile?
     - Do they get your bills right?
     - How long have you been coming here?

Know what you want and need before you get there. Communicate, evaluate, participate, and *communicate*.

4

Close Encounters of the Clinical Kind

— — — — — — — — — — — — — — — — —

Now that you have thought through your personal care expectations and understand how to navigate access systems, what do you think excellent care looks like, and how do you find it? Sometimes people must enter clinical encounters on a leap of faith, while at other times they can enter the encounters with deep and timely research pertaining to credentials, schooling, and treatment options. Whatever your circumstance, you should have a clear vision of what excellent care means to you. Know what enables you to best communicate with your caregiver and what your vision of excellent care looks like.

In urgent situations, we have no time to research. Once the care process is underway and urgency subsides, then there is time for either the patient or patient advocate to become involved with the care process and research, communicate, and participate on an alert and aware level.

In addition to creating the best possible clinical health outcome depending on the patient's health status, excellent care seeks to diminish or eradicate our fear and anxiety. What does excellent care look like?

Although the answer to that question is personal, below are some experiences I believe are examples of excellent care.

Brain or Brawn?

How did my brother and I select a brain surgeon for our mother, who was newly diagnosed with advanced stage brain cancer, in forty-eight hours? We utilized every resource available to us. It was like a SWAT approach. We called everyone we knew who we believed could help support us and provide us with critical data. One friend did numerous Internet searches on Mom's presumed diagnosis and faxed them to us while we were at the hospital. Another friend, a retired medical doctor, said, "Yes, operate." Many others offered support and information relating to anything and everything they believed to be relevant, and of course, a team of clinicians offered more data, in addition to providing the appropriate care and treatment plan to assist with her healing. The retired doctor's wife, a registered nurse, had the words that ultimately were most meaningful for me.

After I described the neurosurgeon who had taken Mom's case, and all of his credentials and schooling, she said, "Well, what I hear is, you have a guy who is midcareer [as she had asked me his approximate age] who is an M.D. and a Ph.D., and I don't hear hesitation in your voice. Do you like him?"

I said, "Yes I do."

She responded, "Then use him." The choice became crystal clear to me at that moment, and it felt right.

The afternoon before Mom's surgery the neurosurgeon first visited with Mom and then came to me and asked if he could do anything for me. Stemming the tide of tears, I said, "I need for you to do a really good job tomorrow." He looked me in the eye and promised he would do his best. His care for Mom was apparent, and that care extended to the rest of our family, too.

We were prepared for any one of the possible outcomes that were presented to us before Mom's frontal lobe was removed. She was in intensive care with tubes and wires running from various parts of her body and to what seemed to be all corners of the room. Her reaction to the intrusion of her central nervous system left her body twitching chaotically.

My brother and I entered her room with the neurosurgeon, and in about sixty seconds the doctor demonstrated that all had gone as well as could be expected. He diminished our fear and anxiety relating to all the frightening visual cues we were receiving.

First, he gave her foot a squeeze and shouted her name. Those actions got her attention, exhibiting to us she knew who she was. We asked about the twitching. He indicated that it was normal and with time should settle down. Then he quite comfortably mentioned, "And that's [the twitching] not bad; I have seen a lot worse." His honesty, confidence, and sincerity, again set our moment-by-moment anxiety to rest.

This neurosurgeon had dispelled every preconceived notion I had about surgeons having no bedside manner. He cared. He cared for Mom for two weeks after her surgery while she lived in Illinois. He cared enough to check in with me genuinely before her surgery. Four-and-a-half months later, he cared enough to phone my home in Vermont and express his condolences for the passing of Mom.

Was this neurosurgeon qualified to perform Mom's surgery? He had all the right degrees from all the right schools, so rationally we expected a good mechanical outcome. The rest of our choice was, in many ways, based on intuition and the ease with which we all communicated. After the surgery Mom returned to more or less the old Mom we knew and loved, and she, too, loved the guy. She had no presurgery recollection of him because of her state of dementia, but most importantly, her communication with him was easy and flowing.

The combination of his demeanor and care left us all with a grounded, honest, well-communicated experience that added confidence in the doctor beyond his neurosurgeon competencies. He was able to diminish fear and anxiety during one of the most stressful events in our lives.

Homeward Bound

Another amazing caregiver was my internist in Vermont. When we moved Mom to Vermont after her brain surgery, I called my internist to see if she would take Mom on as a patient. She agreed. Due to the complexities associated with Mom's health, we agreed to meet with the internist once a week.

The week before Thanksgiving, Mom fell down in the shower. Thankfully, the fall didn't create any serious injuries. The accident was, however, a telltale sign of tumor growth in Mom's head. We attended Mom's weekly appointment with the internist. This appointment concluded differently. The doctor didn't say she would see us in a week, but that *she would be out to see Jayne* at this time next week.

Have you ever had a moment where you believe your ears have disconnected from your brain? I questioned the doctor, "You will come to our house?"

She responded with a warm smile. "Yes, will this time be good for you?" We created a standing time for the doctor to come to our home once a week.

For the remaining weeks of Mom's life, this doctor drove forty minutes one way to my home once a week. I started out believing she was coming to solely care for Mom. After she made several visits, I better understood her role. She was visiting to care for our entire family unit.

In addition to ensuring Mom's comfort, she asked my husband and me how we were holding up, and if we needed anything. Her weekly presence added comfort and diminished our stress and anxiety as Mom's health status changed. She was by our side to communicate with us and answer our questions. The care experience was truly amazing and supportive. She understood Mom's decline would eventually prohibit us from coming to her office, and rather than leave us stranded, she came to us. She cared.

All the Right Stuff

My last example pertains to a physician my husband and I researched, met with, and ultimately selected to perform joint replacement surgery. My husband began his chronic pain journey as a TMJ patient. TMJ, or temporomandibular joint dysfunction, is a condition that erodes the ability for your jaw joint to work properly. The condition causes diminished range of motion and pain. He had been suffering in pain for three-and-a-half years at that juncture and had undergone a multitude of procedures in an attempt to quell the pain.

We had tremendous respect for the physicians in Vermont. However, they hadn't performed but a handful of these joint replacement procedures, and that fact was of concern to us. We asked the Vermont physicians who they felt were the leaders in the field. They suggested two people—a surgeon in New Jersey, and another in Michigan.

We traveled to both places and met with the suggested doctors. Technically, they were both qualified and had performed this procedure with enough volume that my husband and I were comfortable with that data. The reason we chose the surgeon in Michigan (much farther away from where we lived) was because we believed his level of care was greater.

He spent more than two hours with us during our first consultation. He answered all of our questions in a genuine, unrushed fashion. He talked about the reality of the surgery and what it would do to my husband's life from both short- and long-term perspectives. He talked about postoperative physical therapy and posed options. If my husband chose to be self-disciplined and self-motivated, he didn't have to undergo physical therapy. He had examples of patients who had undergone this surgery and gone through physical therapy and others who opted out of physical therapy. He indicated that both sets of patients got to the same place of functionality. He offered rational choices and opportunity to speak with other patients with similar health status. He took the time to get to know us and understand our priorities and lifestyle. In short, he cared.

My husband headed into surgery with confidence that all would go well and with hope that the procedure would end his chronic pain. We knew we had a physician with an expert level of competence on our side, but we also believed he cared about us and our lives. That combination of care made the difference for us. Communication was easy, as was the developing bond of trust.

Art Forms

These three caregivers all share a lively interest in what they do. They are positive and sincere individuals; just like us. They actively participated and created care paths with their patients in the above examples. They integrated the art of medicine into their profession. What I mean by the art of medicine is that the individual's contribution in these cases went beyond the technical skill they acquired from schooling and clinical practice. They are people just like us, but each of them offer their personal gift or their own form of artful medicine to create meaningful, caring relationships and encounters with patients and their family members. As patients, what more can we ask for?

As a patient or patient advocate, when you find the artful clinician it's generally very obvious and your care experience is excellent. Unfortunately, encountering poor care is often equally obvious and typically creates frustration and fear.

Rush Hour

For a two-year period I lived in my hometown county in central New Jersey. Soon after my move, I found myself with a nasty head cold and sinus infection. I hadn't yet procured a primary care physician, so I was at the mercy of the Yellow Pages. Despite my general malaise, I viewed the situation as an opportunity to possibly find a doctor that I liked with whom I could foster a relationship.

I found myself with a same-day afternoon appointment with a female internist who was part of a group about ten minutes from my home. I arrived on time for the appointment and waited only about ten minutes to be transitioned to an exam room. A nurse took all my vital signs, and I described my symptoms to her.

Soon after the nurse departed, another woman, presumably the doctor, swung the door open with such a rush of disorganization that my inner voice said, "This is going to be a nightmare."

She showed little regard for what I might have to say. She didn't ask; she told: "You have an upper respiratory infection." She then proceeded to examine me, checking my eyes, ears, nose, heart, and lungs. Upon listening to my lungs, her level of excitement rose, as though I had stopped breathing.

She said, "Oh, I don't like the sound of those lungs; we *must* get an X-ray."

In all honesty, I felt so crummy I didn't care. I wasn't wheezing. I had run five miles just two days before, but the combination of "the doctor said" and how lousy I felt left me vulnerable to her request. My consumer power, or personal ability to assert myself, was out in the parking lot. Her reaction also planted the seed of fear. I began worrying, "Do I have pneumonia? How could that be?"

Twenty-five minutes later, I was back in the exam room with Dr. No-Listen-but-Talk-a-Lot, and she began writing me one prescription after another—four prescriptions in total. Based on the color of my mucus, all I wanted were antibiotics to clear the infection, but how would she know that? She never asked.

Apparently she was finished, and as she placed one hand on the doorknob, I said, "I have a couple questions." Her body froze, and she emitted a notable sigh. She stood motionless for the first time. Presumably halted by the inconvenience of my words, she waited for me to pose my questions. My first question pertained to the chest X-ray. Was it normal?

"Oh, yes," she responded hastily. "It was fine."

My next question, as I read prescription number two was, "Then why do I need an inhaler?"

She responded, "Just to keep everything open." Her body inched in the direction of the door. I asked my next question.

"What kind of antibiotic did you prescribe? Will it cause my body to get a yeast infection?"

This question incited her most inappropriate behavior. She responded in a condescending tone, "You get *those*?"

"Yes I do, and if I'm going to get one as a side effect of this drug, then I want a prescription for it."

She wrote me another prescription, and I fled the building.

At no point did this clinician take a second to ask about me. At no point did she make an effort to understand what it was I was seeking or needed. Her eye contact with me was minimal, as she was constantly busied with creating diversion and moving on to her next task. Maybe she was Dr. Attention Deficit Disorder.

Reflecting upon this encounter I noted the complete overutilization of services and medications. I left with five prescriptions, three of which I didn't fill. I received an unnecessary chest X-ray, for which I will take some responsibility for complying with the request—but I don't believe I needed the X-ray. I didn't even have a chest-oriented cough. All of my issues were in my sinuses.

In my opinion, the chest X-ray was simply a means to add revenue to the visit. A note to all the clinicians in the audience: My point here is the doctor should have taken the time to explain to me that I had symptoms warranting the X-ray. Had she communicated comprehensively, I wouldn't have reacted and presumed dollars signs were her motivation. Certainly there are instances when a chest X-ray is prescribed due to symptoms the patient may not be aware of.

My thought that the chest X-ray was motivated by money caused the whole visit to take on a different flavor. The doctor's hurried behavior, the extra services, and the perceived unnecessary medications led me to one conclusion about this physician and the group with which she practiced— they cared most about the dollar.

Money is vitally important to the success of good care, and caregivers should be paid very well for their craft. However, providers who place their paycheck at a higher priority than my body and wellness are not the providers I wish to entrust with my health. As a responsible consumer of health care, I did compose a three-and-a-half-page letter outlining my experience with this physician. I mailed the letter to the physician president of the group. I received no response.

Although I state in this case that I neglected to follow doctor's orders and did not fill some of the prescriptions she offered me, I am not advocating on any level that any patient alter a physician's treatment plan or choose not to take the medicine your physician has prescribed for you. Always seek counsel from a physician and communicate your wishes to alter the plan with the physician directly.

RIF—Reading Is Fundamental

When Mom moved to Vermont she needed postoperative care for both her brain surgery and her breast surgery. Before leaving Illinois, I picked up all of Mom's medical records, surgical notes, lab results, slides, and X-rays and made certain the right information got to the right specialists in

Vermont prior to our first visit with each of them. Additionally, I sent each Vermont doctor a twelve-page health summary I wrote that outlined how Mom had come to her current condition.

Our first Vermont visit was with the neurosurgeon. He entered the room completely unprepared. He hadn't read a word of the documentation we provided for him. He had no idea why we were there. His discomfort was palpable as I began asking him all sorts of questions pertaining to the information we forwarded to him via his office manager, Sue. He also hadn't taken the time to return the call to the neurosurgeon in Chicago.

I kept most of my displeasure to myself, as Mom was the patient and therefore "in charge" of the situation. The conclusion of our first visit left Mom disliking this doctor. As you may imagine, Vermont is no bustling hub for neurosurgeons, so with our options limited, we were stuck with the guy.

With time, our relationship with him improved and we came to understand his competencies, but Mom never got over that first encounter. Every time we needed to visit him, and thankfully he wasn't needed as an integral part of her care by that stage, she would be visibly agitated prior to the visit and almost nonparticipative during the visit. He had all the proper degrees and schooling, but his lack of attention to detail, and his visible annoyance by the fact he had to take on another surgeon's patient, caused most of the friction between us and consequently increased our anxiety.

Our first visit to the breast cancer center was no better. Despite my efforts to provide everyone with comprehensive documentation and a summary of Mom's condition, neither the social worker nor the doctor read a word prior to our visit. Instead, they both went into their normal, everyday breast cancer patient routine.

Our purpose for meeting with a breast surgeon was to be certain the drain sites under Mom's arm were healed and were in no need of further attention. An hour and a half after we arrived at the Breast Care Center, we were finally interacting with a physician. He entered the exam room and began curiously attempting to figure out why this woman (Mom) had a dressing on her head. Mom's brain surgery occurred in the front part of her head, and consequently, she was able to retain most of her hair. She did, however, have a healing wound that was still dressed, and it was therefore obvious to an onlooker that this woman had had some procedure performed on her head. He glanced between the chart and Mom and finally asked why we were there.

We described that Mom had just moved to Vermont from Chicago and we needed to be certain her drain site had healed properly as that part of her body was neglected a bit due to the Grade IV brain cancer that was growing in her head.

The doctor quickly examined Mom's incision and indicated that all looked fine. He then directed us to our appointment with the social worker. Wouldn't you hope the doctor might give the social worker a heads–up that her next patient is a breast cancer patient who also is dying of brain cancer?

No luck—in walked the bubbly twenty-something-year-old social worker armed with her Pink Breast Cancer pamphlets and brochures. As we introduced ourselves, I noted that she, too, tried to figure out what the dressing on Mom's head was about. She sat down and began her presentation. At this juncture, I was pretty irritated by the whole episode, but out of respect for Mom, I let the social worker begin her breast cancer spiel.

She covered the breast cancer survivor stories, the support offered by this facility, treatment options, surgery, radiation, chemotherapy, the importance of diet and exercise, and so on. She hadn't even prepared for Mom as a breast cancer patient. Mom was not a *new* breast cancer patient. She had had her treatment, and she didn't need a lecture on breast cancer options.

We let the social worker continue for about ten minutes before we dropped the brain cancer bomb on her, at which point you could see the horror and panic on her face. She realized she hadn't prepared and had presumed we were like every other patient she interacts with all day long. With what little she knew about brain cancer, I think she did manage to deduce the woman (Mom) sitting across the table from her more than likely was terminally ill.

The letter to *that* facility's physician president was seven pages long, detailing access issues, confidentiality problems, and unprepared staff. I got a response from that physician and met with him. The meeting was somewhat disappointing, as he indicated his role at the breast cancer facility was one of appointment, and the fact that he officed across town precluded him from interacting with the day-to-day functions of the clinic. I concluded our meeting by letting him know that I was a thirty-three-year-old woman in need of lifelong breast care, but I would never spend a dime of my health care dollars in his facility. For the remainder of my residence in Vermont, I drove ninety minutes to a university-based breast care center for my annual mammogram.

Surgery 101

When my husband and I chose the surgeon in Michigan for joint replacement surgery, we understood that in addition to the incision made to replace the jaw joint, my husband would also have a incision on his chest where the end of a rib would be removed for a graft and a piece of tissue would be harvested from his buttock to be used in the joint space of his jaw.

Upon completion of the surgery, all went well with my husband's jaw. His other body parts, however, had issues. No one prepared us that the rib harvest could afford the opportunity to puncture a lung, and the surgeon indicated that two grafts had been taken from the buttock area. Apparently a medical student harvested a tissue graft too large and too deep, and when the surgeon got there he had to harvest a smaller, less deep piece of tissue. I never got an answer pertaining to who harvested the rib, a student or our surgeon, but I can venture a guess.

This experience taught us that even though we loved the doctor, and our doctor did a great job as it pertained to the jaw replacement, we couldn't assume that the doctor we loved would be performing every aspect of the surgery. He wasn't even present for the beginning of the procedure, and the students got it less than right, as exhibited by two wounds from the grafts removed from the buttocks. This surgeon did, however, do a good job communicating honestly regarding what went as expected and what did not.

Thankfully, the tissue harvest sites on my husband's buttock were pain free and more of a nuisance because of the daily dressing changes. The lung puncture healed within days, and the jaw replacement was a success. Our overall outcome, despite our moments of added stress due to the unexpected errors, was a positive experience. We would use this surgeon again, because we respected his abilities and appreciated his honest communication under the stressful conditions of the unexpected.

If we were to require his services or the services of any surgeon again, we would require the physician to stipulate in writing that he or she would perform all aspects of the procedure. Minimally, we would require a description of who would be doing what, and we would decide if that course of action were acceptable for us.

You're Fired!

Six months after Mom died we got a call that my father had a "minor" heart attack. I had never heard of a minor heart attack. A heart attack of any magnitude couldn't possibly be minor, but that was the description provided. Dad was taken from his home to the nearest local hospital for treatment of chest pain. Once he was stable, he was moved to a room and admitted to the hospital.

A cardiologist was assigned to him and visited Dad the day of his minor heart attack. For a couple of days, he checked in with my father and ran tests. He indicated that Dad should have angiography, a test in which the coronary arteries or vessels supplying blood to the heart are viewed for blockages.

By then, Dad was feeling better and had regained more of his confidence. He decided that if he needed further care pertaining to his heart, he wanted to be moved to a hospital specializing in heart care.

The next morning, when his assigned cardiologist came by (which, of course, was at a near predawn hour, and no one else from our family was with him), Dad indicated he would like to alter his care path and treatment plan, and be moved to the state's premier heart hospital.

Dad reported that the cardiologist stated reasons why he (Dad) wouldn't want to be moved to what was considered one of the best heart hospitals in the region. When Dad continued to pursue the option to be moved, the cardiologist raised his voice, as he was apparently offended. Dad was simply stating his wishes: he wanted to seek the opinion of another doctor and be moved to a different facility specializing in heart care.

I am not a physician, remember? I am a person just like you. If we apply common sense to the situation, my question is, why would any person, not to mention a person trained in the care of the heart, want to agitate a heart attack patient?! Wouldn't the general goal be to *remove* anxiety and keep the patient calm? The agitated conversation between my father and the cardiologist had nothing to do with healing; it turned into a power struggle between two men. The encounter ended with the cardiologist taking out his prescription pad, writing "You're fired," and tossing the note at my father as he lay in bed.

This cardiologist dramatically "fired" his patient! The termination occurred not because the patient would not take his medications or intended to not pay his bills, but because this patient wanted more and different information. This patient wanted to *participate* in his care and wellness.

This cardiologist made it through medical school and specialist training, but in my opinion, he hasn't left the third grade when it comes to his ability to work with, care for, and communicate with adult human beings. This physician's behavior increased our fear and anxiety, and clearly wasn't a value match for what Dad believed his care should be.

Guardian Angels

As covered in chapter 1, most of my adult health-related experiences have taught me that each patient needs an advocate—a voice. Sometimes patients can be their own advocate and sometimes the patient needs another person to advocate on their behalf. As a little girl, I recall going to the same family doctor until I went to college. This family practitioner provided service to our entire family. He knew us; we all had a relationship with him. When one of us needed care beyond the basic nonurgent office visit, he was there participating in our care and communicating with us and for us. He was the lifelong, steadfast balance to our care experience. We knew him, and we trusted him.

My brother had croup and asthma as a young child. I can recall countless times he was scooped out of the steam-filled bathroom and hauled off to our family doctor's office at 11:00 p.m. I also recall several mornings waking up to find our babysitter watching over me, as my parents and brother had headed to the emergency room, where they were met by our family doctor. This doctor participated in all of the care our family needed. He facilitated the process and communicated with our entire family. He reassured my worried parents, as he reassured me when I had my kidney removed. He was a staple. He was our advocate.

By today's standards, experts might find the concept of the country family doctor who has one partner (and they both know and cover each other's patients) outdated. Looking back, I now see the importance of this physician's role in our lives, and I miss that continuity in the care I find today.

As the glue or advocate for our care experience there was less general worry. A twenty-plus-year relationship spanning generations had proven him honest and caring. We had mutual understanding; we trusted his words and actions.

Whether you are seeking a new doctor or have an established relationship with someone who is a match for your values, let the person know you want this relationship to be long-term. In the case of primary or family care, seek to have the relationship care for your entire family unit. I cannot stress the importance of finding a long-standing relationship and maintaining that relationship for your family unit. The concept may seem silly or old-fashioned when everyone is healthy, but rest assured, *The established, known, and mutually respected relationship with your primary care doctor will prove to be invaluable in a minor crisis, not to mention a major health catastrophe.*

Consider the task of finding and choosing a specialist. If your primary care doctor cannot treat your ailment, he or she may suggest you need a specialist. Wouldn't your comfort level be higher if the person you have known and communicated with for years is suggesting the specialist? Wouldn't that lower your fear and anxiety as it pertains to the person you are about to meet? Wouldn't the odds of the specialist meeting your health and wellness values be greater? You should still interview and research the recommended specialist, but the ease with which you find a match for your situation may be heightened.

Finding a Doctor

When you have the luxury of time to seek out a doctor, I suggest booking a first-visit consultation with the doctor so that you both can experience the interview process. More often than not, the doctor's office will expect your appointment to be for an exam. If your sole purpose for the visit is to consult or interview the doctor, ignore the staff's requests to disrobe. You can politely tell the nurse there is no need to take your vital signs at this stage, as you are here solely to gain understanding and insight into Dr. Smith's care values. If you were feeling bold, you could point out to the nurse you stated your intentions when you booked the appointment, and that you are already disappointed with the communication between staff members. Bring your health record and interview questions, and—as always—be prepared to take notes at the visit.

If you are uncertain what kind of doctor you need, the American Board of Medical Specialties lists physician specialties and subspecialties under the heading "Which Medical Specialist Is for You?" on its website, www.abms.org. The listing is also reproduced in chapter 7.

CREDENTIALS AND EDUCATION PATHS

Generally, doctors follow an education path described in exhibit 4-1.

According to ABMS, the intent of the certification process, as defined by its member boards, *is* "to provide assurance to the public that a certified medical specialist has successfully completed an approved educational program and an evaluation, including an examination process designed to assess the knowledge, experience, and skills requisite to the provisions of high-quality patient care in that specialty."

RESEARCH RESOURCES

How to Tell if Someone Is Board Certified Call the ABMS at 1-866-ASK-ABMS or log on to its website and choose "Who's Certified."

According to the ABMS, most board-certified physicians belong to medical specialty societies. These societies speak to standards and education within their specialty. Full members of these specialty societies are designated as *fellows*. Thus, a physician with the credentials Joe Smith, M.D. F.A.C.S. is a Fellow of the American College of Surgeons and is a board-certified surgeon.

Office of Inspector General The Office of Inspector General (OIG) with the Department of Health and Human Services (HHS) has a database of physicians and organizations that are excluded from federally funded health care programs. The basis for exclusion according to the OIG are "convictions for program-related fraud and patient abuse, licensing board actions and default on Health Education Assistance Loans."

The exclusion does not preclude the physician from practicing medicine. Per the OIG, the effects of an exclusion are the following:

- No payment will be made by any federal health care program for any items or services furnished, ordered, or prescribed by an excluded individual or entity. Federal health care programs include Medicare, Medicaid, and all other plans and programs that provide health benefits funded directly or indirectly by the United States (other than the Federal Employees Health Benefits Plan).

- No program payment will be made for anything that an excluded person furnishes, orders, or prescribes. This payment prohibition applies to the excluded person, anyone who employs or contracts with the excluded person, any hospital or other provider where the excluded person provides services, and anyone else. The exclusion applies regardless of who submits the claims and applies to all administrative and management services furnished by the excluded person.

- There is a limited exception to exclusions for the provision of certain emergency items or services not provided in a hospital emergency room.

Additionally, the exclusions have no bearing on member (the patient) benefits. The exclusion is the ability for the doctor or entity to file a claim

EXHIBIT 4-1 THE PATH TO BECOMING A DOCTOR

LEVEL OF TRAINING	YEARS REQUIRED	TRAINING DETAILS
Undergraduate degree	4 years	Accredited college or university
Medical school	4 years	Doctor of Medicine (M.D.) or Doctor of Osteopathy, (D.O.)
Internship	1 year	First year postmedical school
Residency	3 years	Duration varies by specialty
Fellowship	Varies (1 to 4 years)	Training concentrated on a subspecialty
Licensure	Varies	Licensure is the legal privilege to practice medicine. It is not designed to recognize the skills and knowledge of the trained specialist. License is granted at the state level, and each state has different protocol. The doctor must demonstrate competence to practice medicine in a particular state.
Board certification	Varies	To become board certified by an entity such as the ABMS, the physician generally must follow the education path above and comply with the following: • Complete assessments and documents from the chief pertaining to the individual's performance during residency • Possess an unrestricted license to take the specialty exam • Pass a written exam given by the specialty board • Pass an oral exam conducted by senior specialists in the field (fifteen of the twenty-four ABMS boards require an oral exam)

for reimbursement. An excluded person or facility is precluded from billing a member (the patient) of a federally funded health program directly.

For the purposes of your research, whether your insurance is federally funded or not, the information stored pertaining to your doctor or facility may prove helpful in your care decisions. Check this database even if your insurance plan is not funded by the federal government.

From www.oig.hhs.gov, choose "Exclusions Database." If you discover your doctor or facility is excluded by the OIG, the site will provide an exclusion type and reinstatement information. The exclusion type tells you why the person or entity has been excluded. Reinstatement data will indicate when the person or facility will be reinstated or if they will ever be reinstated.

State Board of Medical Examiners

See chapter 7, or go to www.fsmb.org. The State Board of Medical Examiners will store data pertaining to physicians and their credentials, licensing, disciplinary actions, and so on. The Texas Board of Medical Examiners, for example, provides the following data:

Physician name

License/permit number, date of issue, and expiration

Registration status and date

Disciplinary status and date

Licensure status and date

Mailing address

Primary practice address

Primary type of practice

Secondary type of practice

Education (verification of graduation)

    Program name

    Location

    Type

    Specialty

    Begin and end date

Patient services (sample responses)

    Language translation

    Accessibility to persons with disabilities

    Participation in Medicaid program

Hospital privileges

Specialty board certification

Specialty certification, date, and issuing board

Restrictions and actions

Self-reported disciplinary action by other state medical boards

Criminal history

Malpractice information

    Investigations by the board

    Medical malpractice jury awards

Awards, honors, publications, and academic appointments

The State Board of Medical Examiners will also provide a forum for formal complaints. This venue is the most appropriate entity for formal complaints pertaining to your clinical care performed by a doctor (M.D. or D.O.). Each state will have a process for lodging a complaint.

As a responsible consumer of health care, I encourage the complaint process. On the one hand, if your experience is borne out of a good person having a bad day, then your complaint will cause no harm. If, on the other hand, your complaint is related to incompetence or a pattern of poor care, then your complaint, along with others, will help rectify the care situation for future patients.

Better Business Bureau General complaints are appropriate to send to the Better Business Bureau. You can research local complaints placed with the bureau via its website. Go to the national site and click to your local chapter at www.bbb.org.

Internet The Internet is loaded with data pertaining to health and health care. The American Board of Medical Specialties offers tips for searching and validating information found on the Internet. It indicates that the quality and accuracy of data found on the Internet varies greatly, and "should rarely be accepted without knowing that the source of the information is credible." The board suggests that the website content come from a reputable peer-reviewed medical journal or that other qualified health professionals have reviewed the material. If you are unsure as to the credibility of the information found on the Internet, print out the material and ask your doctor for his or her opinion. Among other websites, the ABMS suggests www.mayoclinic.org as a credible website for health-related information.

NURSING CREDENTIALS

Similar to doctors, nurses have state boards governing licensure. See www.howtogetthehealthcareyouwant.com for a complete state-by-state listing. The State Board of Nursing organization will typically host a database of licensed nurses as well as serve as a venue for formal complaints.

Licensure Nurses are licensed as advanced practice nurses, registered nurses (RNs), or as licensed practical/vocational nurses (LPNs/LVNs). Nurses must be licensed in the state where they work. After graduation, they must pass a license examination to become a licensed nurse. To obtain an RN, the nurse must successfully complete the two- to three-year associate degree level or higher. Formal education programs for nurses are listed as follows. These descriptions are supplied by www.nursingsociety.org.

- **Bachelor of Science in Nursing (BSN)** A four-year program offered at colleges and universities prepares nurses to practice across all health care settings. BSN graduates have the greatest opportunity for advancement.
- **Associate Degree in Nursing (ADN)** A two- to three-year program offered at junior and community colleges. An associate's degree trains and prepares nurses to provide direct patient care in numerous settings.
- **Licensed practical nurse (LPN)** In Texas and California, these nurses are called licensed vocational nurses (LVN). These nurses care for the sick, injured, convalescent, and disabled patients under the direction of

physicians and registered nurses. They provide basic care, taking vital signs, temperature, blood pressure, and pulse, and assist with bathing patients, monitoring catheters, and applying dressings.

- **Hospital diploma** A two- to three-year hospital-based nursing program affords nurses the ability to deliver direct patient care in a variety of environments.

Continuing Education Although only mandated in some states, all nurses are expected to keep current with nursing practice and advance as health professionals after graduation. Nurses can also pursue advanced degrees in the profession.

Advanced Nursing Degrees

- **Master's degree (MSN)** Master's degree programs prepare nurses for more independent roles such as nurse practitioner, clinical nurse specialist, nurse-midwife, nurse anesthetist, or nurse psychotherapist. Nurses with a master's degree serve as expert clinicians, in faculty roles, and may specialize in geriatrics, community health, administration, nursing management, and other areas.

- **Doctoral degree (Ph.D., Ed.D., DNS)** Doctoral programs prepare nurses to assume leadership roles within the profession, conduct research that impacts nursing practice and health care, and teach at colleges and universities. Doctorally prepared nurses serve as health system executives, nursing school deans, researchers, and senior policy analysts.

- **Postdoctoral programs** Postdoctoral programs provide advanced research training for nurses who hold doctoral degrees.

Certification RNs can become certified in their specialties as a measure of clinical competence. For the different types of certification available, go to the American Nurses Association website, www.nursingworld.org, and search for certifications.

Questions to Consider While Evaluating Clinicians

Suggestions for evaluation and data collection regardless of the role the clinician is playing in your treatment are listed in exhibit 4-2. You could add some or all of these questions and their answers to your standard care expectations list.

EXHIBIT 4-2 EVALUATING CLINICIANS

PERSONAL

1. Years in practice?
2. Medical school graduate of _____?
3. Internship performed at _____?
4. Undergraduate degree in _____ from where _____?
5. Why did you become a _____ doctor?
6. How do you prepare for exams or procedures? Will you read chart notes and documentation I send to you? Will you read the documentation other doctors send to you before I arrive for my appointments?
7. What was the most exciting thing you learned recently that pertains to your career as a _____ doctor?
8. If we mutually agree that this relationship is a match, will you be committed to my care until I am well (or for my lifetime, in the case of primary or family care)?
9. Have you ever had your hospital privileges revoked? If yes, where and why?
10. How would you feel if I were to need a second or third opinion pertaining to my health? How would you facilitate my request?
11. Considering I track my medical history and will require my doctor(s) to read my history and share their charting with me, how did this doctor respond when I explained that? How will he/she share my chart notes with me? Via fax? USPS? secure e-mail? If I am in the hospital, how will I receive my medical record notes each day?
12. Understanding we are all humans and humans make mistakes, can you, in general terms, describe a medical mistake you made and what you did to rectify the situation?
13. Can you have three patients with my similar health status contact me as references?
14. Who will call me with test results? Will it be you, the doctor, or do you delegate that to a nurse? Can I request that you call me with the results? Will you mail or fax my results to me? How soon after the tests can I expect my results?
15. If I am in the hospital, are you willing to book an appointment (or perform your rounds) at a mutually agreed upon time (e.g., not 5:45 a.m.)?

COMMUNICATION AND REACTIONS

1. Was my initial reaction to this person a perception of a caring individual?
2. Did the person introduce himself or herself in a comfortable, approachable, confident way?
3. How did the conversation flow? Was the person a good listener? Did he/she maintain good eye contact? Did I understand what the person was saying?
4. Did the person ask me well-rounded questions? Did the questions expand beyond the scope of the one section of my body that is ailing? In a primary care situation, did the questions include my entire body, my emotional state, my family, and my life?
5. Did I leave feeling comfortable with this person? Could I trust this person with my life?
6. Is there some sort of bond with the person? Do I feel safe? Is the communication easy and flowing? If I didn't understand something, did the person take the time to ensure that I understood?
7. Can this doctor comply with most or all of my standard expectations as outlined in chapter 1?
8. What does my intuition (or gut) tell me about this person?
9. Did this person do what he or she said would be done?

INSURANCE AND FINANCE

1. Is this doctor part of my insurance network?
2. Does this doctor plan to remain part of my insurance network? If this doctor changes or cancels contracts with insurance companies on a regular basis then you will either need to incur greater cost to continue care with this provider or seek care from another provider (thus, losing the relationship).
3. Does this doctor have organized business practices?
4. What are the billing and collections policies?

Evaluating Health Care Facilities

Because I have only one kidney, I have my blood and urine checked every six months. The last round of testing called for my standard blood work, a urinalysis, and a twenty-four-hour urine test. My nephrologist's office was completely inept in describing what I needed to do for the twenty-four-hour urine test—and that is a story for another day. I did, however, manage to glean that I needed to go to the lab and "pick up a jug."

When I got to the lab, there was no one in the waiting room. I signed in on their noncompliant sign-in sheet and gave the person behind the glass window my requisition. After writing my first initial and last name with a Sharpie on a cup, she handed it to me and pointed to the restroom. I entered the restroom to find the toilet had overflowed and was clearly still clogged. Immediately, I assessed the rest of the bathroom and concluded that I have visited many gas station ladies' rooms that were cleaner than this facility.

I exited the restroom and interrupted the conversation at the check-in desk with, "Do you know your toilet has overflowed?"

The woman hastily headed to the bathroom, looked at the toilet, and engaged her problem-solving abilities. The first thing she noticed, that I quite frankly missed, was someone had used a paper towel and left it in the basket of unused wipes. She quickly snatched a clean paper towel and removed the used paper towel from the basket and threw all of it in the waste can.

My brain was screaming, "What about the wipes—aren't they contaminated, too?" I said nothing.

She told me that this was their only restroom. I had no desire to use this nonfunctioning restroom, so we agreed that I would drop off the urine sample when I dropped off the twenty-four-hour sample. A phlebotomist drew my blood, and I left the facility, jug in hand.

The following Monday, I returned with a jug full of twenty-four hours' worth of my urine. The test required I emptied my bladder in the morning, twenty-four hours after I first began collecting the sample. That meant I would have to donate the smaller sample of urine for the other urinalysis when I got to the lab. Knowing the bathroom was gross, I figured I would get through the experience with a significant level of denial, because I really just wanted to drop off the jug, head to work, and be done.

I arrived at the lab, signed in, gave the woman the jug and my requisition, and headed for the bathroom. There was no real change in status of the restroom. The toilet had not recently overflowed, but the general filth remained. The bathroom was outfitted with one of those little doors that allow you to leave your urine sample for the lab, which resides on the other side of the wall. I opened the little door to leave my cup and found about five other samples resting on a urine-stained paper towel. My first reaction was general disgust. Then an even more horrifying thought crept in. It was about 7:30 a.m. The lab opened at 7:00 a.m. When I got there, no one was in the waiting room. Could those samples have been left from the day before? Disgusting!

Behind the reception area, I also noticed test tubes of blood piled on a filing cabinet. The sight of twenty or so blood-filled vials haphazardly left on the filing cabinet lying on their sides created an uneasy feeling for me. I think my reaction related to some sort of physical privacy violation. The specimens of other human beings are not my business, I felt awkward seeing them in disarray. Then I was saddened by the idea that presumably my blood had been carelessly left there as well. There was no sanctity associated with the sight.

As I was leaving, the woman behind the counter stopped and said they needed to collect blood from me. I told her, "No, I did that last week." She said, "We need blood to go with the twenty-four-hour urine." So I got stuck in the arm again.

Why couldn't the lab have told me it needed blood with the twenty-four-hour urine? I would have waited and completed *all* of my blood work at one time with one stick of the needle. Besides avoiding having my body invaded twice, I would have saved the cost of a syringe and the time it took to draw the blood and process the specimen. This facility was a disgrace.

When most of us think of a health care facility we think hospital or doctor's office. However, a plethora of facilities require licensure and accreditation, ranging from nursing homes, outpatient surgery centers, rehabilitation facilities, imaging centers, and of course doctor's offices and hospitals. The Joint Commission on Accreditation of Healthcare Organizations (JCAHO) continuously strives "to improve the safety and quality of care provided to the public through the provision of health care accreditation and related services that support performance improvement in health care organizations."

JCAHO is an independent, not-for-profit organization established more than fifty years ago and is governed by a board that includes physicians, nurses, and consumers. Joint Commission sets the standards by which health care quality is measured in the Unites States and around the world.

JCAHO evaluates the quality and safety of care for more than fifteen thousand health care organizations. To maintain and earn accreditation, organizations must have an extensive on-site review by a team of Joint Commission health care professionals at least once every three years. The purpose of the review is to evaluate an organization's performance in areas that affect care. Accreditation may then be awarded based on how well the organization met Joint Commission standards.

A list of Joint Commission accredited organizations and their survey results are posted in the "Quality Check" section of the Joint Commission website, www.jcaho.org. You can also call Joint Commission's customer service department directly at (630) 792-5800 for additional information.

The website has a simple search function to guide you by category of facility (i.e., hospital, outpatient surgery center, etc.) and your zip code. In addition to access to the quality reports, the site functionality offers the ability to compare one facility with another. Exhibit 4-3 shows a sample comparison.

The JCAHO process for accreditation begins with the facility requesting the survey. Therefore, just because a facility is not accredited doesn't mean the facility has issues to be concerned about. You could, however, ask your doctor why he or she has chosen not to seek accreditation. The lab I referenced earlier is not accredited by JCAHO.

The Internet offers health care consumers many venues to support health-related encounters. You can research providers and facilities, and when necessary, lodge complaints. As a patient receiving care, utilize your advocate(s) to maintain your voice and communication when need be and to help you be an astute communicator. Communicate about everything. Communicate, participate, evaluate, and communicate.

EXHIBIT 4-3 EXCERPT FROM WWW.JCAHO.ORG

HOSPITAL COMPARISON

FUNCTION	HEALTH CARE ORGANIZATION	
	Hospital A	Hospital B
National Patient Safety Goals Met	A	A

NATIONAL QUALITY IMPROVEMENT GOALS

	Hospital A	Hospital B
Heart Attack Care	A	A
Heart Failure Care	A	B
Pneumonia Care	B	A $_1$
Pregnancy Care	B $_1$	E $_2$

This measure is part of the Hospital Quality Alliance. This measure can also be viewed at www.cms.hhs.gov.

1 - The measure or measure set is not reported.
2 - The measure set does not have an overall result.
3 - The number of patients is not enough for comparison purposes.
4 - The measure results are not displayed.
5 - The organization scored above 90% but was below most other organizations.
6 - The measure results are not statistically valid.
7 - The measure results are based on a sample of patients.
8 - The number of months with measure data is below the reporting requirement.

KEY

A This organization achieved best possible results.
B This organization's performance is above the performance of most Joint Commission–accredited organizations.
C This organization's performance is similar to the performance of most Joint Commission–accredited organizations.
D This organization's performance is below the performance of most Joint Commission–accredited organizations.
E This measure is not applicable for this organization.
F Not displayed.

5

Cash Management— Will It Hurt?

— — — — — — — — — — — — — — —

Buy the best insurance you can afford. Maintaining your physical health is a large task when illness threatens your lifestyle. You don't want to add the burden of worry and stress relating to finances while in a health crisis. Health insurance is the single most important insurance purchase you make.

Generally, you are looking for a plan that fits your budget and offers the most flexibility and coverage regarding your care choices. Flexibility is important for the reasons we have discussed in the previous chapters. As discussed in chapter 1, a good health care experience is related to matching up your personal goals and expectations with those of your caregivers. Hence, flexibility is an important aspect of your insurance plan so you can find the caregivers who meet your needs, expectations, and values.

The adage "You get what you pay for," may not necessarily relate to care provided. There have been many studies indicating the ability for one to pay for care has no direct correlation to the quality of care dispensed and received. You can, however, buy flexibility, which increases your options, and this may, in fact, add to your peace of mind.

The cost of the twisted ankle case study outlined in chapter 3 is approximately as follows:

First office visit	$100.00
Soft brace	$35.00
Ankle X-ray	$300.00
Follow-up office visit	$75.00
	$510.00

If the injury were more serious, possibly a break or a tear requiring the attention of a specialist and some physical therapy, the tab would have run up into the $3,000 zone.

First office visit	$100.00
Soft brace	$35.00
Ankle X-ray	$300.00
Specialist visit	$150.00
MRI of ankle	$2,100.00
Cast	$200.00
Physical therapy	$150.00
Physical therapy	$60.00
Physical therapy	$60.00
Physical therapy	$60.00
Physical therapy	$60.00
Physical therapy	$60.00
Follow-up office visit with specialist	$85.00
	$3,420.00

The cost associated with caring for a simple twisted ankle, which is something that could happen to any of us at any time, exhibits why health insurance is important.

Many of us are easily confused by terminology relating to health insurance. The variety of options that insurance companies present can send anyone's head spinning in confusion and worry pertaining to cost and benefit coverage. Many people feel like they choose health insurance from a place of uncertainty and hope, rather than one of confidence, knowing, and clarity. The key to confidence and clarity is understanding to the best of your ability what's *not* covered.

Just like any other large purchase, research and investigation are warranted. Who goes out and purchases a new stereo, plasma TV, or new car without researching cost, performance, and how the product fits with one's life? Purchasing health insurance may not feel like a large purchase because your employer may contribute to your premium, or as a relatively healthy person, you don't often use your health insurance. Health insurance is one of life's most important choices. When evaluating health insurance, focus not on health, but disaster. Think about the worst possible health crisis you can imagine and then attempt to calculate, in conjunction with your health benefits, what your annual health care costs would be.

Discovering health care–related costs when you are in the middle of the health crisis only adds to the stress of the situation. Because purchasing health insurance is one of the largest, most important purchases we make, it is important that we understand how it works with relation to our care and our wallet. The more you know about your health insurance exclusions (what's not covered) and the rules associated with accessing care (preauthorization and prior notice), the safer your personal finances remain.

Identifying the Best Insurance You Can Afford

How do you know how much insurance you can afford? Let's first examine the financial components of health insurance that affect your personal finances.

PREMIUM

The premium is the cost to purchase the insurance. If you are employed and your employer offers health insurance for you and your family, your employer is paying the premium for your insurance. In some cases, employers will pay a portion of the premium and the employee makes a contribution to the premium via a payroll deduction. That contribution is your portion of the premium or the expense associated with purchasing the insurance.

If you are insured by a government-funded plan such as Medicare or Medicaid, there are sometimes premiums for additional coverage. For example, if you are a Medicare recipient and you wish to purchase Medicare B coverage for outpatient services, or purchase a Medicare supplemental insurance, the cost associated with either of those purchases is the premium for such coverage.

DEDUCTIBLE

The deductible is an annual portion of your care for which you are financially responsible. When your deductible has been met your insurance begins paying for services. This assumes, of course, that the service is covered by your plan. If you have an annual $250 deductible, you will pay $250 of your dollars toward your care before insurance will begin paying for care. Knowing when your plan year begins and ends is important so you can prepare for the deductible cost at the beginning of the plan year.

CO-PAY

Co-pay pertains to the portion of the bill for which the patient is responsible, provided the service is covered by your plan. If, for example, your insurance plan requires the patient pay a $25 co-payment for primary care office visits but your plan excludes chiropractic services, then you, the patient, are responsible for paying for the entire chiropractic visit—for example, $45.

COINSURANCE

Coinsurance is different from co-payments. If your plan requires 20 percent coinsurance after deductible, you must pay your annual deductible and will then be responsible for 20 percent of the *allowed*, or contracted, rate for the services covered by your health insurance.

Your insurance company and doctor or facility can have a contract. If a doctor's office visit costs $100 and your doctor and your insurance company have agreed the expected reimbursement for your office visit is $80 and your plan states you have a 20 percent coinsurance, then your insurance is going to pay $64 (or 80 percent of the *allowed* or contracted amount of $80) and you are responsible for 20 percent of the $80, or $16.

The combination of your coinsurance and the insurance company's payment sums to $80, or the expected reimbursement per the contract between the provider, the insurance company. Please note that when you buy insurance you are contractually agreeing to pay all deductibles, co-payments and coinsurance to your providers. If you neglect to pay your portion, there is typically language in the certificate of coverage that allows the insurance company to terminate your coverage.

You may be beginning to understand why it's difficult to find a person working in health care who can tell you exactly how much something is going to cost. Are you also beginning to understand that the billed charge, or the amount the doctor or hospital lists as owed (in this example, $100) is irrelevant to what the doctor or facility actually expects to get paid?

If the doctor agrees to a rate for a particular service, and he or she knows the expected reimbursement is $80, then whether the charge is $100 or $1,000,000 is irrelevant, and only matters if you don't have insurance. I describe options for those who are uninsured and underinsured later in this chapter.

As already stated, the insurance company requires that the patient pay coinsurance. If the doctor or facility has a contract and they have agreed upon an expected reimbursement, that expectation includes the patient portion. Essentially, the policy holder (patient or subscriber to insurance) has a contractual obligation to pay co-payments, deductibles, and coinsurance. Count on the requirement to pay your coinsurance and deductible, not the ability of your doctor or hospital to write off your balance. Your certificate of coverage may have language stating failure to pay coinsurance can result in termination of your health insurance coverage. If you are insured by a government payor such as Medicare or Medicaid, the provider of services (i.e., the doctor or hospital) are required by law to collect your coinsurance, co-payments, and deductibles unless, you, the patient can demonstrate financial hardship.

OUT-OF-POCKET MAXIMUM

In general, the out-of-pocket maximum is the maximum amount of coinsurance/co-payments a patient will make in one plan year. If the plan's out-of-pocket maximum is $2,000, then the most you will expect to pay for care your plan covers over the course of one year is $2,000. Some plans include your deductible and co-payments in the out-of-pocket maximum and some plans do not. Your certificate of coverage will delineate what counts toward your out-of-pocket maximum.

PRECERTIFICATION/PREAUTHORIZATION

Insurance companies attempting to control cost and ensure patients receive appropriate care based on health status may require some services be *preauthorized*. Typically, the burden of obtaining authorization is the patient's responsibility. Preauthorization of service does not guarantee payment for service.

NONCOVERED SERVICES

Services not covered by your plan or services deemed not medically necessary are wholly the patient's responsibility and do not count toward deductibles or out-of-pocket maximums. Additionally, these services do not fall under the contract between your doctor and the insurance company so there is no allowable or contractual adjustment. In the previous example, you would be responsible for the entire charge or the entire $100.

The Bottom Line

What is my annual health care liability?

Today's health insurance climate offers thousands of different health plan options to consumers and employers. I cannot possibly present all of them. I intend to point out what to examine when shopping or choosing your health insurance. The material presented in this section is not true for all health insurance plans and programs, but it provides a general synopsis of how a typical plan is described to a consumer by the insurance company and how to evaluate a plan description.

Most health insurance plans have *in-network* providers and facilities, meaning the insurance company and the doctor or hospital have a contract delineating reimbursement. If your insurance only provides benefits when you see an in-network provider, then you have chosen a plan that is pretty much in control of the providers and facilities you can visit if you want your services covered.

Steer is a strong word, and insurance companies react to the word negatively, but that is essentially what a network is meant to do. If a patient's health insurance cost is lower to see in-network or contracted providers, then more often than not patients are going to seek care from those in-network providers. The insurance company uses the financial enticement to get the patient to see one of the in-network providers.

Insurance companies may refute allegations relating to steering patients with the fact that they have large networks with broad scopes encompassing entire communities and covering all specialties of care. Therefore, patients can choose from a wide spectrum of providers. The size of the network is important and may offer patients varieties of options. If, however, you have chosen an in-network *only* plan and that one doctor your uncle swears is the best is not in the network, the fees associated with seeing Uncle Bill's favorite doctor will not be paid by your insurance.

As a consumer of care, be very aware of which providers are in the plan's network and what geographical area the network services. Utilizing the insurance company's website will provide the most current list of in-network providers. Be aware that sometimes the website is incorrectly loaded. *I suggest you print the screen and maintain the document in your health record.*

If the insurance company should happen to deny your claim as out of net-work, you would then have proof that the insurance company advertised a provider or facility as in-network on the day you received your service.

Some insurance companies will provide you with a booklet listing all in-network providers. Keep the booklet, as it is a document important for your plan evaluation. The booklet, however, tends to get outdated quickly, so use the website or call the insurance company's customer service num-ber if you need clarity.

Your doctor can terminate his or her agreement with an insurance plan at any time, you could accept a new job, or you could become ill on vaca-tion or at college. Any of these events could affect your personal financial resources. If any of these situations occur, you may need to pay a larger portion (or the entire portion) of your care or be forced or *steered* toward creating new care relationships with providers and facilities that are in your health plan's network. Remember the important discussion in chapter 4: you want your primary doctor to be by your side for the long haul. So find out if your doctor intends to remain contracted with your insurance plan for the long haul.

If, for example, you find yourself admitted to a non-network hospital because you fell off your roof and the ambulance took you to the closest hospital, you may find yourself being moved from that hospital to an in-network hospital, provided your condition is stable. If the doctor you've known and loved is no longer in your insurance plan's network, you will need to create a new care relationship with a new doctor or else pay for your care in its entirety from the doctor your want to keep.

The same situations could unfold if you change jobs or if your employer changes plans. If your plan changes and the new plan has different in-net-work providers, your choices are to pay more to preserve and maintain the relationship with the provider you know and love, switch to new caregivers, or convince your current provider to contract with your new plan. Even if your current provider agrees to contract with your new plan, realize that process will take some time, and during that time, should you need care, you will pay more for the care you receive from that provider.

Budget Analysis

THERE IS MATH ON THIS TEST

Employers may provide a choice to employees. Employees may be offered an HMO (in-network only) or PPO (in- and out-of-network options). Your human resource department or insurance broker may give you a summary that looks like exhibit 5-1.

SAMPLE BENEFIT SUMMARY

Ascertaining your annual out-of-pocket cost is the first step to plan evaluation. My first budget example pertains to a relatively healthy single person who works. This person's employer pays the premium. The person intends to use only "in-network" providers and facilities.

Example 1: HMO coverage for a single person

STEP ONE: GATHER ALL HEALTH-RELATED COSTS	
Premium contribution (per paycheck payroll deduction)	$0.00
Annual deductible	$0.00
In-network out-of-pocket maximum	$2,000.00
Last year's medication cost plus 20%	$120.00

STEP TWO: CALCULATE THE ANNUALIZED COST	
Annual premium expense ($0 × 26 pay periods)	$0.00
In-network out-of-pocket maximum	$2,000.00
Last year's medication cost plus 20%	$120.00
Total annual maximum cost	$2,120.00

NOTE: The out-of-pocket maximum includes co-payments and deductibles, but does not include costs for medications.

EXHIBIT 5-1 SUMMARY COMPARISON OF INSURANCE PLANS

	HMO	PPO NETWORK	PPO NON-NETWORK
ANNUAL DEDUCTIBLE	$0 per covered person per calendar year.	$250 per covered person per calendar year, not to exceed $500 for all covered persons in a family.	$500 per covered person per calendar year, not to exceed $1,000 for all covered persons in a family.
OUT-OF-POCKET MAXIMUM (OOPM)	$1,500 per covered person per calendar year, not to exceed $3,000 for all covered persons in a family.	$2,000 per covered person per calendar year, not to exceed $4,000 for all covered persons in a family.	$4,000 per covered person per calendar year, not to exceed $8,000 for all covered persons in a family.
OUT-OF-NETWORK BENEFITS	None	When covered health services are received from non-network providers, eligible expenses are determined based on either: • Fee(s) that are negotiated with the provider • 110 percent of the published rates allowed by Medicare for the same or similar service • 50 percent of the billed charge • An existing fee schedule developed by the insurance company Note: If care is received from a non-network physician, facility, or other health care professional you will incur greater financial expense compared to an in-network provider. Your plan only pays a portion of those charges, and it is your responsibility to pay the remainder. You are required to pay the amount that exceeds the allowable amount, which could be significant, and that amount does not apply to the out-of-pocket maximum. Ask the non-network physician or health care professional about billed charges before you receive care.	
MAXIMUM POLICY BENEFIT	Unlimited	No maximum policy benefit	$1,000,000 per covered person.

This person has an annual health care liability of $2,120 *for services covered by his insurance plan*. In many regards, the budget is that simple. Should a health crisis strike, and this person seeks care within the insurance company's predetermined network of providers and facilities, and the care is provided per the terms of the certificate of coverage, and medications cost the same or slightly more than last year, he should not pay more than $2,120 in one plan year for his health care.

If the goal is to remove stress relating to finances during episodes of illness, then maintain a savings account to cover your annual health care liability. Maintaining a savings account for your care will ensure you have enough funds to cover your annual out-of-pocket *possible* expense. If you were to become seriously ill, and you were the person in example 1, the annual health care–related expense liability would be $2,120.

You could choose to maintain twice the annual liability to cover the current year of your illness and therefore afford yourself the time to restock funds the following year once you are well. Should your illness become of a chronic or debilitating nature, you would also have time and resources to locate other care options, such as free care or less expensive care.

Example 2: HMO coverage for a family This example is similar to example 1. However, instead of coverage for just one person, coverage is provided for the employee, spouse, and three children. This family also commits to utilize in-network providers only. Easy calculation!

STEP ONE: GATHER ALL HEALTH-RELATED COSTS	
Premium contribution (per paycheck payroll deduction)	$420.98
Annual deductible	$250.00
In-network out-of-pocket maximum	$4,000.00
Last year's medication cost plus 20%	$820.00
STEP TWO: CALCULATE THE ANNUALIZED COST	
Annual premium expense ($420.98 × 26 pay periods)	$10,945.48
In-network out-of-pocket maximum	$4,000.00
Last year's medication cost plus 20%	$820.00
Total annual maximum cost	$15,765.48

NOTE: The out-of-pocket maximum includes co-payments and deductibles, but does not include costs for medications.

Example 3: PPO coverage for a single person This example is similar to example 1: a healthy individual gets her insurance from her employer, but she wants the flexibility to see providers outside the network.

STEP ONE: GATHER ALL HEALTH-RELATED COSTS	
Premium contribution (per paycheck payroll deduction)	$24.30
Annual deductible	$250.00
In-network out-of-pocket maximum	$2,000.00
Out-of-network out-of-pocket maximum	$4,000.00
STEP TWO: CALCULATE THE ANNUALIZED COST	
Annual premium expense ($24.30 × 26 pay periods)	$631.80
In-network out-of-pocket maximum	$2,000.00
Out-of-network out-of-pocket maximum	$4,000.00
Last year's medication cost plus 20%	$120.00
Total annual maximum cost	$6,751.80

NOTE: Budget the cost of both the in- and out-of-network out-of-pocket maximums in the event you choose to use both. A point to paying extra for this plan is to have the flexibility to go out of network. The out-of-pocket maximum includes co-payments and deductibles, but does not include costs for medications.

Example 4: PPO coverage for a family If the family in example 2 wanted the flexibility to utilize in- and out-of-network providers, its maximum annual out-of-pocket potential cost would be as follows.

STEP ONE: GATHER ALL HEALTH-RELATED COSTS	
Premium contribution (per paycheck payroll deduction)	$478.81
Annual deductible	$250.00
In-network out-of-pocket maximum	$4,000.00
Out-of-network out-of-pocket maximum	$8,000.00
Last year's medication cost plus 20%	$820.00

NOTE: The out-of-pocket maximum includes co-payments and deductibles, but does not include costs for medications.

STEP TWO: CALCULATE THE ANNUALIZED COST	
Annual premium expense ($478.81 × 26 pay periods)	$12,449.06
In-network out-of-pocket maximum	$4,000.00
Out-of-network out-of-pocket maximum	$8,000.00
Last year's medication cost plus 20%	$820.00
Total annual maximum cost	$25,269.06

As you can see, flexibility adds cost to the equation. Ensuring that the doctors and facilities you intend to utilize are in-network will have a cost savings effect for your budget. These four examples offer a basic, simple way to begin to understand your annual worst-case cost liability. As we continue the plan evaluation process, we may uncover other costs that relate to you and your situation, and those costs should be added to your budget.

The "in-network only" model is typically referred to as an HMO, or health maintenance organization, and is usually cheaper. The option that affords the patient the opportunity to be seen either in-network or out-of-network is typically called a PPO, or preferred provider organization.

If we are healthy when we evaluate insurance, cost is usually one of our first concerns. The important factors relating to cost are premium, out-of-pocket maximum, and your best guesstimate pertaining to medication co-payments expended in prior years. If you have saved to cover your out-of-pocket maximum liability, and you have budgeted for your monthly premium, then if you become seriously ill during the course of the year you should have most of the cash to pay for your portion without added worry relating to money.

Our rational brain tends to prevail in analytical situations. Never in our wildest dreams do we believe serious illness will strike. Nor can we fathom what that disaster will really mean to our lives. Choosing insurance based on dollars can be a simple, rational process. Many of us want to believe that the cheapest option is the best option. It's easy to convince yourself you are immortal, infallible, and the healthiest person walking the planet. "Why save? Nothing bad ever happens to me. Why spend the money on the PPO plan that allows me to see both in- and out-of-network providers? I won't need my insurance."

On a cool fall morning when I lived in New Jersey, I received a call from an old friend in Vermont. We hadn't spoken in months, so I was excited to hear from her. Her voice quaked as she said, "Dave is really sick, can you help me?"

Dave, her husband, was in his late thirties, a master-degreed professional working for one of our nation's largest employers. She called because she knew I had survived many health-related encounters with both my mom and husband. Dave's condition was life-threatening cancer. Her questions for me were not at all financially oriented, nor did I expect them to be. As a family unit, they were a financially stable, well-educated couple with one child. Presumably, they had excellent health benefits.

Our discussion focused on getting Dave the right care and how to manage their lives during this period of crisis. Then I said, "You will certainly seek care outside Vermont, won't you? Mayo, Sloan Kettering, or even Dartmouth may be options." After a long pause, she responded, "We can't. It would bankrupt us."

The story ends positively. Dave received care in Vermont, and more than three years later, he enjoys his work, life, and family. The care he received in Vermont was successful. However, the added burden of being limited to a relatively small community of providers weighed heavily on the entire family during the initial period of discovery and research relating to treatment options for what is a very uncommon cancer. They stepped though discussions pertaining to bankruptcy (obtaining care outside the network) and living or dying (perceived limitations of care inside the network). Dave chose an in-network-only HMO plan from his employer, and that choice limited his care to the community in which he lived.

If you are choosing an in-network-only HMO plan, understand that your options for care may be broad, but are limited. That statement doesn't mean you won't receive care benefits, nor does it mean you will receive substandard care. Choosing an in-network-only HMO product means you have less say in who provides your care if you expect your insurance benefits to cover the care.

What's Not Covered

The budget we have just outlined *only* pertains to items *covered* by your insurance. What about the stuff that's not covered? What about the stuff that doesn't count toward your out-of-pocket maximum? The next step of evaluation is to read your certificate of coverage and learn what's not covered. The subsequent pages will lead you through a sample evaluation of exclusions and noncovered benefits.

Begin with your certificate of coverage. Ask your HR department or your insurance broker for a copy. Read the entire document, but start with the chapter called "Exclusions" and read every word. As you read, note the exclusions that matter to you. List your questions, and seek clarity for any language that is vague. Although you can't predict the future, you can budget more accurately if you know you are likely to need services that are not covered or that do not count toward your out-of-pocket maximum.

Usually you will find a blanket statement indicating the plan may not pay for benefits for any services, treatments, items, or supplies described in these sections *even if the service is recommended or prescribed by a physician and it is the only treatment available for your condition.*

I don't know a healthy person who could actually put dollars relating to liability next to those words, but the message is most certainly an important one to understand and contemplate.

Once you have digested the "Exclusions" chapter of the certificate of coverage, you need to move on to the "Covered Benefits" section. In this section read with an eye for more noncovered *services* and read with an eye for flexibility. Even though this is the benefit coverage section, read between the lines and you will discover other excluded items that could potentially affect you wallet. Note the types of services that require authorization and prior notification.

For example, in the section outlining covered benefits under dental services, dental services are only covered in the case of an accident and if the initial contact with the physician or dentist occurred within seventy-two hours of the accident.

The following text comes from one company's "Covered Benefits" section in its certificate of coverage.

> Benefits are available only for treatment of a sound, natural
> tooth. A virgin or unrestored tooth, or a tooth that has no decay,
> no filling on more than two surfaces, no gum disease associated
> with bone loss, no root canal therapy, is not a dental implant and
> functions normally in chewing and speech.[2]

These words would eliminate coverage for some of the teeth in my mouth, and if I were prone to barroom brawls I would add funds to my annual out-of-pocket liability budget, because the likelihood I would need to utilize dental care not covered by my health insurance would be high.

Exhibit 5-2 is a comparison of certificates of coverage for HMO (in-network) and PPO (in- and out-of-network plan) exclusions found in both the exclusion section, "What's Not Covered" and the benefit section, "What Is Covered," of the certificate of coverage.

The first column of exhibit 5-2 depicts an HMO certificate of coverage, while the second column represents the certificate of coverage for a PPO. The third column lists thoughts, questions, and differences. The fourth and fifth columns note if either of the PPO or HMO terms will increase the annual cost of care ($ indicates a slight increase and $$$$ a significant increase). The last column is used to indicate your preference, HMO or PPO.

Exhibit 5-2 is a simple Excel spreadsheet. You can easily use this format to evaluate your own certificate of coverage.

EXHIBIT 5-2 PLAN COMPARISON EXAMPLE

HMO IN-NETWORK ONLY[3]	PPO IN- AND OUT-OF-NETWORK [4]	CONTROL/FLEXIBILITY CONCERNS/QUESTIONS	PPO COST	HMO COST	PATIENT PREFERENCE
DENTAL EXCLUSIONS Dental X-rays, supplies and appliances, and all associated expenses, including hospitalizations and anesthesia. The only exceptions to this are for any of the following (meaning the following would be covered): the direct treatment of acute traumatic injury, cancer, or cleft palate.	Same as HMO	What is acute traumatic injury? Could that mean getting punched in the face and losing a tooth? Or does that mean falling down a flight of stairs and breaking several teeth? Or does that mean loss of teeth due to smashing into a windshield? If I were punched in the face and lost a tooth, I would consider that acute and traumatic, but would the health plan? Call and ask for clarity.			NONE
DENTAL BENEFITS Dental services are only covered in the case of an accident and if the initial contact with the physician or dentist occurred within seventy-two hours of the accident. Benefits are available only for treatment of a sound, natural tooth. A virgin or unrestored tooth, or a tooth that has no decay, no filling on more than two surfaces, no gum disease associated with bone loss, no root canal therapy, is not a dental implant, and functions normally in chewing and speech.	Same as HMO except when using an out-of-network provider. Patient must notify insurance company when utilizing out-of-network providers or facilities. Failure to provide notification will result in a 50 percent reduction in benefits.	That language would eliminate coverage for some of the teeth in my mouth. Does the PPO reduction in benefits apply to my out-of-pocket maximum?	$	$	

EXHIBIT 5-2 PLAN COMPARISON EXAMPLE

HMO IN-NETWORK ONLY[3]	PPO IN- AND OUT-OF-NETWORK [4]	CONTROL/FLEXIBILITY CONCERNS/QUESTIONS	PPO COST	HMO COST	PATIENT PREFERENCE
DIABETES TREATMENT BENEFITS No comment regarding, supplies, medications, and equipment	All supplies, including medications and equipment for the control of diabetes, shall be dispensed as written, including brand name products, unless substitution is approved by the physician or practitioner who issues the written order.	PPO benefits appear to be richer. Call to see if what is covered under PPO is covered under HMO.		$	PPO

EXHIBIT 5-2 PLAN COMPARISON EXAMPLE

HMO IN-NETWORK ONLY[3]	PPO IN- AND OUT-OF-NETWORK [4]	CONTROL/FLEXIBILITY CONCERNS/QUESTIONS	PPO COST	HMO COST	PATIENT PREFERENCE
DIABETES EQUIPMENT BENEFITS Insulin pumps and associated appurtenances Insulin infusion devices Podiatric appliances	Insulin pumps, both external and implantable, and associated appurtenances, which include insulin infusion devices, batteries, skin preparation items, adhesive supplies, infusion sets, insulin cartridges, durable and disposable devices to assist in the injection of insulin, and other required disposable supplies. Benefits are included for repairs and necessary maintenance of insulin pumps that are otherwise not provided for under warranty or purchase agreement. Benefits are also included for maintenance of insulin pumps (neither of which shall exceed the purchase price of a similar replacement pump). Podiatric appliances (including up to two pairs of therapeutic footwear per year for the prevention of complications associated with diabetes.	No mention of insulin infusion devices for PPO plan			

EXHIBIT 5-2 PLAN COMPARISON EXAMPLE

HMO IN-NETWORK ONLY[3]	PPO IN- AND OUT-OF-NETWORK [4]	CONTROL/FLEXIBILITY CONCERNS/QUESTIONS	PPO COST	HMO COST	PATIENT PREFERENCE
DIABETES SUPPLY BENEFITS Visual reading and urine test strips Injection aids Syringes	Visual reading and urine test strips and tablets that test for glucose, ketones, and protein Injection aids, including devices used to assist with insulin injection and needless systems Insulin syringes				
DRUGS Noninjectable medications given in a physician's office except as required in an emergency	Same as HMO	What constitutes an emergency? Do you have to be in the emergency room of the hospital for Xanax to be covered? Call and ask for clarity.	$	$	
COMFORT AND CONVENIENCE EXCLUSIONS Batteries and battery charges	Batteries and charges, except that batteries for insulin pumps are a covered health service for covered persons with diabetes	See questions under Diabetes Coverage.	$		PPO

EXHIBIT 5-2 PLAN COMPARISON EXAMPLE

HMO IN-NETWORK ONLY[3]	PPO IN- AND OUT-OF-NETWORK [4]	CONTROL/FLEXIBILITY CONCERNS/QUESTIONS	PPO COST	HMO COST	PATIENT PREFERENCE
EXPERIMENTAL, INVESTIGATIONAL, OR UNPROVEN SERVICE Experimental, investigational, and unproven services are excluded. The fact that an experimental, investigational, or unproven service treatment, device, or pharmacological regimen is the only available treatment for a particular condition will not result in benefits if the procedure is considered to be experimental, investigational, or unproven in the treatment of that particular condition.	Same as HMO	The language is very vague. Who determines what is experimental, investigational, or unproven? Ask for a current list of treatments, services, supplies, and devices that fall into this category.			
FOOT CARE EXCLUSIONS Shoe orthotics	Shoe orthotics, except as described as a covered health service for covered persons with diabetes	See diabetes questions and coverages.		$	

EXHIBIT 5-2 PLAN COMPARISON EXAMPLE

HMO IN-NETWORK ONLY[3]	PPO IN- AND OUT-OF-NETWORK[4]	CONTROL/FLEXIBILITY CONCERNS/QUESTIONS	PPO COST	HMO COST	PATIENT PREFERENCE
MENTAL HEALTH AND SUBSTANCE ABUSE EXCLUSIONS

Services performed in connection with conditions not classified in the current edition of the *Diagnostic and Statistical Manual of the American Psychiatric Association.*
Services for mental health and substance abuse that extend beyond the period necessary for short-term evaluation, diagnosis, treatment, or crisis intervention
Treatment for mental illnesses that will not substantially improve beyond the current level of functioning, or for conditions not subject to favorable modification or management according to generally accepted standards of psychiatric cares as determined by the mental health/substance abuse designee
Residential treatment services except as specifically described as a benefit in Mental Health Services | Services performed in connection with conditions not classified in the current edition of the *Diagnostic and Statistical Manual of the American Psychiatric Association*
Services for mental health and substance abuse that extend beyond the period necessary for short-term evaluation, diagnosis, treatment, or crisis intervention
Treatment for mental illnesses that will not substantially improve beyond the current level of functioning, or for conditions not subject to favorable modification or management according to generally accepted standards of psychiatric cares as determined by the mental health/substance abuse designee
Residential treatment services
Services utilizing methadone treatment as maintenance, L.A.A.M. (1-alpha-Acetyl-Methodol), Cyclazocine, or their equivalents | Mental health and substance abuse categories tend to follow different rules than the rest of the benefits offered. If you had an inkling you or a family member were going to need to use your mental health and or substance abuse benefit, a trip to the American Psychiatric Association's website may be in order, www.psych.org.
How long is short-term? Who determines the length of period?

Wow, that sounds like if you aren't going to get better, they just give up. Call and ask for clarity. | | | |

EXHIBIT 5-2 PLAN COMPARISON EXAMPLE

HMO IN-NETWORK ONLY[3]	PPO IN- AND OUT-OF-NETWORK [4]	CONTROL/FLEXIBILITY CONCERNS/QUESTIONS	PPO COST	HMO COST	PATIENT PREFERENCE
OUTPATIENT MENTAL HEALTH			$		PPO
Services are limited to thirty visits per year. Referrals to a mental health provider are at the sole discretion of the mental health/substance abuse designee, who is responsible for coordinating all of your care. Authorization is required. Without authorization, you will be responsible for paying all charges and no benefits will be paid, unless services are received as a result of an emergency. Contact the mental health/substance abuse designee regarding benefits for outpatient services. Please remember that you must call and get authorization to receive these benefits in advance of any treatment through the mental health/substance abuse designee. Without authorization, you will be responsible for paying all charges and no benefits will be paid, unless services are received as a result of an emergency. Outpatient co-payment is $25 per visit, $10 per group visit, and counts toward out-of-pocket maximum.	Any combination of network and non-network benefits for mental health services and/or substance abuse services is limited to thirty visits per calendar year. No authorization required In-network co-payment: Outpatient co-payment is $25 per visit, $10 per group visit, and does not count toward out-of-pocket maximum. Out-of-network co-payment is 30 percent of eligible expenses and counts toward out-of-pocket maximum.	HMO—Not only should you call and get clarification as to what is covered, but this aspect of coverage appears to be bureaucratic and controlling. Additionally, we need clarification on what is an emergency and what level of training does the mental health/substance abuse designee have. Do you, the patient, meet with that person? How does confidentiality work?			

EXHIBIT 5-2 PLAN COMPARISON EXAMPLE

HMO IN-NETWORK ONLY[3]	PPO IN- AND OUT-OF-NETWORK [4]	CONTROL/FLEXIBILITY CONCERNS/QUESTIONS	PPO COST	HMO COST	PATIENT PREFERENCE
PREEXISTING CONDITION No clause	Benefits for the treatment of a preexisting condition are excluded until the date you have had continuous creditable coverage (under the policy or under any other plan) for twelve months.	If you have had a recent lapse in coverage, the PPO preexisting condition clause could create enormous additional cost if you have a preexisting condition. If you really want PPO coverage, a suggestion would be to go on HMO for the first year and then switch to PPO. At then end of the year you would be able to switch to PPO coverage and not worry about the added cost of the pre-existing condition.	$$$		
REPRODUCTION EXCLUSIONS Health services and associated expenses for infertility treatments that are determined to be experimental, investigational, or unproven services. In vitro fertilization, gamete intrafallopian transfer (GIFT) procedures, and zygote intrafallopian transfer (ZIFT) procedures, and any related prescription drug treatment to create a pregnancy. Donor ovum and semen and related costs, including collection and preparation.	Health services and associated expenses for infertility treatments	PPO—What services? Ask for a list of known experimental, investigational, or unproven services.	$$$		HMO

EXHIBIT 5-2 PLAN COMPARISON EXAMPLE

HMO IN-NETWORK ONLY[3]	PPO IN- AND OUT-OF-NETWORK[4]	CONTROL/FLEXIBILITY CONCERNS/QUESTIONS	PPO COST	HMO COST	PATIENT PREFERENCE
TRANSPLANT EXCLUSIONS Health services connected with the removal of an organ or tissue from you for purposes of a transplant to another person. (Donor costs for removal are payable for a transplant through the organ recipient's benefits under the contract.) Any solid organ transplant that is performed as a treatment for cancer Transplant services that are not performed at a designated facility	Health services connected with the removal of an organ or tissue from you for purposes of a transplant to another person. (Donor costs for removal are payable for a transplant through the organ recipient's benefits under the contract.) Any solid organ transplant that is performed as a treatment for cancer. No designated facility requirement, but a $30,000 maximum per transplant for out-of-network services	If I am going to donate my kidney to my brother, this insurance company says my brother's insurance company is going to cover me for my services; now how would they know that? Investigation needed. Additionally, reading that statement made me want to go to the section describing what is covered to see if this plan states it covers the donating party in the case that I am the recipient. There was no language to that effect in the transplant section for covered benefits. I would most certainly call for clarity. The PPO does not, however, indicate the recipients insurance will pay for the donor's costs; the plan limits the out-of-network benefits to $30,000. I would investigate the benefit further.	$	$$$	

EXHIBIT 5-2 PLAN COMPARISON EXAMPLE

HMO IN-NETWORK ONLY[3]	PPO IN- AND OUT-OF-NETWORK [4]	CONTROL/FLEXIBILITY CONCERNS/QUESTIONS	PPO COST	HMO COST	PATIENT PREFERENCE
TRAVEL EXCLUSIONS Health services provided in a foreign country, unless required as emergency health services travel or transportation expenses, even though prescribed by a physician. Some travel expenses related to covered transplantation services may be reimbursed at our discretion.	Same as HMO	What constitutes emergency health services? If you are in Germany and your kidney stone flares up, is that an emergency? How do you plan a budget around "reimbursed at our discretion?" Call and seek clarity.	$	$	None
ALL OTHER EXCLUSIONS Health services received as an act of war Health services received after the date your coverage under the policy ends Health services for which you have no legal responsibility to pay In the event that a non-network provider waives co-payments and/or the annual deductible for a particular health service, no benefits are provided for the health service for which the co-payments and/or annual deductible are waived Charges in excess of eligible expenses or in excess of a specified limitation	Same as HMO	Remember out-of-network billed charges can exceed the insurance company's eligible reimbursement amount and you could wind up paying the difference. This is the sentence that prevents/discourages the provider from waiving or adjusting off the patient responsibility. Ask the insurance company for its allowable rates.		$$$	

EXHIBIT 5-2 PLAN COMPARISON EXAMPLE

HMO IN-NETWORK ONLY[3]	PPO IN- AND OUT-OF-NETWORK [4]	CONTROL/FLEXIBILITY CONCERNS/QUESTIONS	PPO COST	HMO COST	PATIENT PREFERENCE
DURABLE MEDICAL EQUIPMENT BENEFITS

If more than one piece of durable medical equipment can meet your functional needs, benefits are available only for the most cost-effective piece of equipment.
We provide benefits only for a single purchase (including repair/replacement) of a type of durable medical equipment once every three calendar years. We decide if the equipment will be purchased or rented. You must purchase or rent durable medical equipment from the vendor we identify. | Same as HMO
PPO requires notification for items that cost more than $1,000. If you don't notify your insurance company, benefits will be reduced to 50 percent of eligible expense; however, the reduction in benefits will not exceed $500. | The HMO plan sounds like they are buying the cheapest and expecting it to last three years. If you want something different or wish to utilize a different vendor, you pay.
If you are going to choose the PPO plan and you are seriously ill (i.e., exceeding your out-of-pocket maximum), the reduction in benefits should you neglect to inform the payor really doesn't matter if it counts toward the out-of-pocket maximum. Does it or doesn't it? Call for clarification. | $$ | $$ | |
| EYE EXAMINATIONS – BENEFITS

Covered every other year
In-network co-payment is $25 per visit and does count toward out-of-pocket maximum. | Covered every other year.
In-network co-payment is $25 per visit and does not count toward out-of-pocket maximum.
Out of network co-payment is 30 percent of eligible charges and does count toward out-of-pocket maximum. | I wear contacts and have to go to the eye doctor every year. I would budget for that extra visit if I were on the PPO plan. | $ | $$ | |

EXHIBIT 5-2 PLAN COMPARISON EXAMPLE

HMO IN-NETWORK ONLY[3]	PPO IN- AND OUT-OF-NETWORK [4]	CONTROL/FLEXIBILITY CONCERNS/QUESTIONS	PPO COST	HMO COST	PATIENT PREFERENCE
HOME HEALTH CARE—BENEFITS Home health care is not delivered for the purpose of assisting with activities of daily living, including but not limited to dressing, feeding, bathing, or transferring from a bed to a chair. No limit is listed.	Same as HMO Out of network co-payment is 30 percent eligible expenses and does count toward the annual out-of-pocket maximum. Any combination of network and non-network benefits is limited to sixty visits per calendar year. One visit equals four hours of skilled care services. Notification is required five days before receiving services for non-network benefits. Failure to provide notification will result in a reduction of benefits by 50 percent not to exceed $500.	The words "but not limited to" should prompt a call. I would want more clarity on what exact conditions are covered for home health care. Is there a limit for HMO?		$$	
PROSTHETIC DEVICES BENEFITS If more than one prosthetic device can meet our functional needs, benefits are available only for the most cost-effective prosthetic device.	Same as HMO	No flexibility			

EXHIBIT 5-2 PLAN COMPARISON EXAMPLE

HMO IN-NETWORK ONLY[3]	PPO IN- AND OUT-OF-NETWORK[4]	CONTROL/FLEXIBILITY CONCERNS/QUESTIONS	PPO COST	HMO COST	PATIENT PREFERENCE
RECONSTRUCTIVE PROCEDURES BENEFITS Cosmetic procedures are excluded from coverage. Procedures that correct an anatomical con-genital anomaly without improving or restoring physiologic function are considered cosmetic procedures. The fact that the covered person may suffer psychological consequences or social avoidance behavior as a result of an injury, sickness, or congenital anomaly does not classify surgery or other procedures done to relieve such consequences or behavior as a reconstructive procedure.	Same as HMO Notification required. Failure to notify the insurance company will result in a reduced benefit of 50 percent eligible expenses; however, the reduction in benefits will not exceed $500.				
SKILLED NURSING FACILITY/INPATIENT REHABILITATION FACILITY SERVICES Benefits are limited to sixty days per calendar year.		PPO has no limit? Call for clarity.	$		
TEMPOROMANDIBULAR JOINT SERVICES Benefits include diagnostic or surgical treatment required as a result of accident, trauma, con-genital defect, development defect, or pathology. Benefits are not provided for any dental services. Dental splints are excluded.	Same as HMO		$	$	

EXHIBIT 5-2 PLAN COMPARISON EXAMPLE

HMO IN-NETWORK ONLY[3]	PPO IN- AND OUT-OF-NETWORK [4]	CONTROL/FLEXIBILITY CONCERNS/QUESTIONS	PPO COST	HMO COST	PATIENT PREFERENCE
PRESCRIPTION DRUGS BENEFITS	Same as HMO	That means there is no annual maximum for your co-payments related to medications. The sky is the limit.	$$$	$$$	
The amount you pay in co-payments or for any noncovered drug product will not be included in calculating any out-of-pocket maximum. You are responsible for paying 100 percent of the cost (the amount the pharmacy charges you).					
SPINAL TREATMENT	Same as HMO	That means there is no annual maximum for your co-payments related to these services.	$	$	
Spinal treatment for detection or correction (by manual or mechanical means) of subluxation(s) in the body to remove nerve interference or its effects is not included in calculating any out-of-pocket maximums.					

EXHIBIT 5-2 PLAN COMPARISON EXAMPLE

HMO IN-NETWORK ONLY[3]	PPO IN- AND OUT-OF-NETWORK [4]	CONTROL/FLEXIBILITY CONCERNS/QUESTIONS	PPO COST	HMO COST	PATIENT PREFERENCE
EMERGENCY HEALTH SERVICES BENEFITS	Co-payment is $100 per visit and does not count toward out-of-pocket maximum.			$	HMO
Co-payment is $50 per visit, which counts toward the out-of-pocket maximum.	If admitted into a non-network hospital as a result of an emergency, you must notify the insurance company within forty-eight hours or as soon as reasonable possible.				
	If you don't notify the company, benefits for the non-network hospital inpatient stay will be reduced to 50 percent of eligible expenses. However, the reduction in benefits will not exceed $500. Benefits will not be reduced for the outpatient emergency health services.				
HOSPITAL INPATIENT STAY BENEFITS	In-network same as HMO	PPO: Does the reduction in benefits relating to authorization count toward my out-of-pocket maximum?			
Co-payment is 10 percent and counts toward out-of-pocket maximum.	Out-of-network co-payment is 30 percent and counts toward out-of-pocket maximum.				
	Notification required for out-of-network facilities. Benefits for the non-network hospital inpatient stay will be reduced to 50 percent of eligible expenses; however, the reduction in benefits will not exceed $500.				

EXHIBIT 5-2 PLAN COMPARISON EXAMPLE

HMO IN-NETWORK ONLY[3]	PPO IN- AND OUT-OF-NETWORK [4]	CONTROL/FLEXIBILITY CONCERNS/QUESTIONS	PPO COST	HMO COST	PATIENT PREFERENCE
PHYSICIAN OFFICE SERVICES	In-network benefits do not count toward out-of-pocket maximum. Non-network benefits do count toward out-of-pocket maximum.		$$		
REHABILITATION SERVICES OUTPATIENT THERAPY BENEFITS In-network co-payment counts toward out-of-pocket maximum. No limitations stated. Benefits are available for rehabilitation services that, in the opinion of the covered person's network physician, are expected to restore a covered person to the previous level of functioning (not to exceed activities of daily living). Benefits for rehabilitation services are not available for services that are expected to provide a higher level of functioning than the covered person previously possessed. For a physically disabled person, treatment goals may include maintenance of functioning or prevention of or slowing of further deterioration.	In-network co-payment does not count toward out-of-pocket maximum. Any combination of network and non-network benefits is limited as follows: Twenty visits of physical therapy per calendar year Twenty visits of occupational therapy per calendar year Twenty visits of speech therapy and or hearing therapy per calendar year Twenty visits of pulmonary rehabilitation therapy per calendar year Thirty-six visits of cardiac rehabilitation therapy per calendar year	HMO: Are there limits like the PPO benefit?	$$$		

EXHIBIT 5-2 PLAN COMPARISON EXAMPLE

HMO IN-NETWORK ONLY[3]	PPO IN- AND OUT-OF-NETWORK [4]	CONTROL/FLEXIBILITY CONCERNS/QUESTIONS	PPO COST	HMO COST	PATIENT PREFERENCE
OUT-OF-NETWORK BENEFITS None	When covered health services are received from non-network providers, eligible expenses are determined based on either fee(s) that are negotiated with the provider, 110 percent of the published rates allowed by Medicare for the same or similar service, 50 percent of the billed charge, or a fee schedule that we develop. If care is received from a non-network physician, facility, or other health care professional you will incur greater financial expense compared to an in-network provider. Your plan only pays a portion of those charges and it is your responsibility to pay the remainder. You are required to pay the amount that exceeds the allowable amount, which could be significant, and that amount does not apply to the out-of-pocket maximum. We recommend you ask the non-network physician or health care professional about their billed charges before you receive care.	If you wish to know what the Medicare published rates are for the current year, they can be found in the Federal Register in the health and safety section, search for [current year] Medicare fees. Note: this is not light reading. 50 percent of the billed charge leaves you at risk for the provider or facility whose charge is inappropriately high. You can use Medicare rates as your guide. A doctor's fee would be considered normal if it were approximately 2.5 to 3 times Medicare's current fee. The patient is responsible for paying the difference between the billed charge and plan payments. Request the fee schedule the insurance company has developed and ask that it be amended to your certificate of coverage each year. With this plan example, having out-of-network benefits doesn't mean that those benefits will have an equal effect on your wallet.		$$$$$	

Once you have evaluated the exclusions listed in the "Exclusions" chapter and uncovered the exclusions listed in the "Covered Benefits" chapter, you need to refigure your annual out-of-pocket maximum to the best of your ability. If you believe some of your care in the coming year falls under the exclusions, pay close attention and do your best to estimate your cost. If you see an acupuncturist and her services are excluded from your coverage, then, you need to add your acupuncture visits to the budget.

None of us can predict the future, but the goal is to create as much financial reality as you can. Once you have the numbers, the answers to your questions, and plan comparison in front of you, then you can make an informed, more confident decision about how to spend and budget your health care dollars.

I would also suggest you keep your research focused on your certificate of coverage. The certificate of coverage is the legal binding document describing your coverage terms. Seek to get your questions answered in writing, and if you feel skeptical about an answer, pay attention to that feeling and ask a different person at the insurance company the same question to see if you get the same answer.

The certificate of coverage will also provide you with the official steps to complain and file appeals. Navigating a large insurance company with an issue or question that is important to you can be frustrating. I suggest initially following the outline for complaints and appeals described in your certificate of coverage. If that procedure doesn't prove to be fruitful, your next stop is your human resource department for those who receive coverage via their employer.

If you are buying your own insurance, validate that your insurance agent is credible and operating in good faith. Contact your state department of insurance and make sure the agent and the company you are working with is licensed. When purchasing the policy make certain your check is made out to the insurance company, not the agent or the agent's company. Maintain receipts for all premium payments made.

The National Association of Insurance Commissioners (NAIC) offers the following tips to avoid fraudulent plans (www.NAIC.org):

- Call your state department of insurance and validate that the agent and the insurance company are registered with the state.

- Fraudulent plans are most often sold through direct-mail solicitations or over the Internet, so be especially wary when responding to these types of solicitations.

- If a policy costs far less than what other companies are charging, this could be a warning sign. It is a good idea to comparison shop, but if a policy is significantly cheaper, beware.

- Beware of an agent or company that refuses to provide proof of state licensure; insists on cash payments or automatic withdrawal; states this is a "one time deal" or "last chance for special savings"; and boasts that the coverage is available to anyone, regardless of history or risk.

The National Committee for Quality Assurance (NCQA) is a private, not-for-profit organization. NCQA assesses and reports on the quality of the nation's managed care plans. The organization evaluates quality via accreditation, the Health Plan Employer Data and Information Set (HEDIS), and comprehensive member surveys. The NCQA website can be found at www.healthchoices.org.

According to the website, NCQA evaluates how well the health plan provides it members with access to care with good customer service. Are there enough primary care providers? Are there enough specialists to serve the number of people subscribing to the plan? Does the plan have quality providers? NCQA evaluates the health plan's ability to ensure each doctor is licensed and trained to practice medicine and whether the subscribers are happy with the doctors and facilities in the plan.

The NCQA evaluates the health plan's ability to assist its members with maintaining health and wellness and preventing illness. When a plan member becomes ill, the NCQA is interested in what activities the health plan deploys to assist people to recover from illness. For example, how does the health plan evaluate new medical procedures, drugs, and devices? If the member's illness is chronic, the NCQA cares about how the health plan proactively assists with chronic conditions. Does the health plan, for example, provide annual eye exams for diabetic patients?

For each of the categories the NCQA rates, the website uses a simple star rating system to understand how the health plan is doing in a particular category. The NCQA also offers an accreditation for HMOs, PPOs, and managed behavioral health care organizations (MBHOs).

If you and your insurance company are in disagreement after the grievance process and working through your human resource department, the next step is to file a formal complaint and grievance with your state department of insurance. If dissatisfaction continues, then pursue mediation, arbitration, and, lastly, litigation.

How to Use Health Savings Accounts

Funding an employer-sponsored flexible spending account (FSA) is a way to reduce current-year out-of-pocket health care–related costs through tax deduction savings. Funds contributed to the FSA are pretax and can be used to cover co-payments, coinsurance, and other noncovered health-related expenses as defined by the plan.

The primary disadvantage to an FSA is the money left unused at the end of the plan year is no longer yours. If you fund your FSA with your calculated out-of-pocket annual liability and disaster does *not* strike, you no longer have those funds for the following year—hence, the suggestion for a personal savings account for funds relating to the *possibility* of illness.

If you have the option to utilize an FSA, trend your past health-related expenses. If you were to review the past three years, took an average of expenses and added a small percentage for inflation, you may come up with a safe and reasonable amount to allocate for your FSA.

If for example, your family spent on average $800 on co-payments, prescriptions, eye glasses, etc., over the past three years and you believe the likelihood of maintaining that level of health care utilization will remain about the same, then fund your FSA with at least $800 and reap the tax benefit associated with the FSA.

If you fund the FSA with what your average annual out-of-pocket health-related expenditures were *that contributed to your plan's* annual out-of-pocket maximum, then you could lessen or subtract that dollar amount from your out-of-pocket annual liability personal savings account. Conversely, if you are funding your FSA to purchase services not covered by your insurance, then do not subtract that sum from your personal savings account budget. (See exhibit 5-4)

Health savings accounts, or HSAs, offer tax relief for the consumer portion of health-related costs as well. An HSA is a tax-exempt trust or custodial account that is set up with a qualified HSA trustee to pay or reimburse certain medical expenses. Consumers must qualify for an HSA account by choosing a particular type of health insurance.

The qualifications needed to open an HSA account are that the patient is enrolled in a high-deductible health plan (HDHP) as defined by the Internal Revenue Service (IRS). See publication 969 at www.irs.gov for current-year limits and definitions for qualifications.

The primary benefit to an HSA is that the patient can claim a tax deduction for contributions made by the patient or another party (provided the other party is not the patient's employer), the contributions remain in your account from year to year until they are used by the patient, the interest or other earnings on the assets in the account are tax free, distributions may be tax free if you pay qualified medical expenses with the distribution. Last, the HSA is portable, meaning if the patient changes employers the account and the money in it remains with the patient.

In general, qualified medical expenses include amounts paid for doctor's fees, prescription and nonprescription medicines, and necessary hospital services not paid for by insurance. Qualified medical expenses are those incurred by the patient or the patient's spouse, or by dependents on the account owner's tax return. See IRS publication 502 for detailed qualified medical expenses (www.irs.gov). Exhibit 5-3 compares your liabilities using an HMO versus a PPO when savings accounts are not included. Exhibit 5-4 shows how the comparisons break out when savings accounts are part of the mix.

EXHIBIT 5-3 PERSONAL SAVINGS ACCOUNT AND COVERAGE DECISION
WORKSHEET (with no health savings account and no flexible spending account)

HMO (IN-NETWORK ONLY)		PPO (IN- AND OUT-OF-NETWORK)	
Annual premium	$_____	Annual premium	$_____
Out-of-pocket maximum	$_____	Out-of-pocket maximum in-network	$_____
Noncovered services, treatments, medications, or supplies	$_____	Out-of-pocket maximum out-of-network	$_____
Annual liability (or budgeted contribution to your personal savings account)	$_____	Noncovered services, treatments, medications, or supplies	$_____
		Annual liability (or budgeted contribution to your personal savings account)	$_____
HMO ADVANTAGES		PPO ADVANTAGES	
_____		_____	
HMO DISADVANTAGES		PPO DISADVANTAGES	
_____		_____	

Government Payers: How to Know What's Covered

The Centers of Medicare and Medicaid website is www.cms.gov. From that site you can choose either Medicare or Medicaid under the consumer information tab. If you are a Medicare recipient, the current-year Medicare manual will suffice as your certificate of coverage and can also be found at www.cms.gov.

If you don't have Internet access, you can reach the Centers for Medicare and Medicaid Services via telephone at 877-267-2323 or by writing to Centers for Medicare & Medicaid Services, 7500 Security Boulevard, Baltimore, MD 21244-1850.

EXHIBIT 5-4 PERSONAL SAVINGS ACCOUNT AND INSURANCE PLAN DECISION
WORKSHEET (with employer-sponsored flexible spending account)

HMO (IN-NETWORK ONLY)		PPO (IN- AND OUT-OF-NETWORK)	
Annual premium	$_____	Annual premium	$_____
Out-of-pocket maximum	$_____	Out-of-pocket maximum in-network	$_____
Noncovered services, treatments, medications, or supplies	$_____	Out-of-pocket maximum out-of-network	$_____
Minus FSA contribution	$(_____)	Noncovered services, treatments, medications, or supplies	$_____
Annual liability (or budgeted contribution to your personal savings account)	$_____	Minus FSA contribution	$(_____)
		Annual liability (or budgeted contribution to your personal savings account)	$_____
HMO ADVANTAGES		PPO ADVANTAGES	
HMO DISADVANTAGES		PPO DISADVANTAGES	

Utilizing the current-year Medicare manual will help you step through the same budget process that was previously described. You may also want the publication called "Your Medicare Benefits" (CMS pub. No. 10116), found at www.medicare.gov/publications.

Medicaid and Children's Health Insurance (CHIP) are state-run programs providing health benefits to the indigent and financially needy. If you believe you may be eligible for Medicaid or CHIP, the same website, www.cms.gov, provides an overview of benefits and eligibility information. The site will redirect you to your state Medicaid program.

Additionally, www.cms.gov provides a synopsis of federally mandated Medicaid-covered benefits. Your state will be able to provide a comprehensive description of benefits and exclusions.

Billing and Collections

Billing and reimbursement mistakes can occur. Determination of your claim's payment or denial is based on the services provided to you and why those services were provided, meaning your diagnosis or medical necessity. Additionally, the provider of service must send the insurance company all of the correct data elements relating to you and the care you received. A mistake on your bill doesn't necessarily indicate fraud. A basic clerical error can occur at any step in the billing process. If you receive a denial from your insurance company and you believe the claim should have been paid, call both your insurance company and the doctor or hospital.

A common misperception patients maintain is that the hospital or facility is one-stop shopping. In other words, you will receive one bill from the hospital and that's it. Not true. The hospital is one entity, but all of the doctors (i.e., anesthesiologist, surgeon, radiologist, pathologist) who provided you with services while you were at the hospital will send you their bills, in addition to the hospital's or facility's invoice. The doctors work for themselves, and their billing will not be included in the hospital or facility's invoice. Even if you go to a hospital on an outpatient basis, expect to receive a bill from that facility and from the doctor who read your test results or provided your service.

When you believe a billing error has occurred, don't be overly surprised when the insurance company tells you the error is on the part of the provider and the provider faults the insurance company. First verify with your doctor and/or facility all the services for which they are billing. Were all of those services performed? Then ask what diagnosis they are using for billing purposes, and make sure it is correct. Last, verify all of the other data elements they are using to submit your claim:

Patient's name

Patient's date of birth

Patient's address

Patient's telephone

Patient's Social Security number

Subscriber's name (person who supplies the patient with insurance coverage)

Subscriber's date of birth

Subscriber's address

Subscriber's telephone

Policy number

Group number

Insurance company name

Insurance company claim address

If you still believe a billing error has occurred, call customer service at your insurance company and ask the person to pull up your denied claim. Make the company tell you what was billed (i.e., what service or procedure was performed) and why (diagnosis). Does the insurance company's story match the provider's story?

If the stories match and the provider billed what the insurance company denied and you agree the services and diagnosis are correct, but you believe the claim should be paid, then you need to work through the appeal and complaint process with your insurance company.

Your certificate of coverage will provide detailed instructions pertaining to the claim appeal process and the complaint process. As you work through the complaint process, be prepared for a slow-moving bureaucracy. Tell the provider or facility that you are appealing the claim with the insurance company and ask the provider to hold your account from further collection efforts until you receive resolution. They may request you pay a small good-faith payment each month while you await determination, or you may be required to pay in full.

If the insurance company has no record of your claim, then return to the provider of service and ask to review all the data elements submitted on your claim. Odds are, the provider has incorrect information relating to your group number, policy number, or claims address.

If you believe your complaint should be lodged with the state department of insurance, the National Association of Insurance Commissioners (NAIC) website, www.naic.org, will direct you to your state's department for the purpose of logging a complaint. The state department of insurance website also maintains a complaint scorecard for insurance companies operating in each state. The scorecard may assist with determining if your insurance company has a problem servicing its patient base.

Health care fraud occurs when a provider of service bills for something that wasn't performed. If you believe your provider is systematically and purposefully creating fraudulent claims, you can report instances of alleged fraud to your state department of insurance on the NAIC website. You can report Medicare fraud to 1-800-447-8477, or go to www.oig.hhs.gov.

Uninsured and Underinsured

What should you do if you can't afford to pay your health-related bills? Ask for assistance. If you can't afford to pay your coinsurance and deductibles, ask the provider if it has a financial assistance program. Most providers offer services at a discount if the patient can demonstrate need. Ask what programs are available.

If you believe you qualify for government assistance, seek the assistance of a social worker. If you have access to the Internet, go to www.cms.hhs.gov and search for Medicaid and CHIP.

6

Creating and Maintaining Your Own Health Record

Why take the time to create and maintain your own health record? The reality of today's health care delivery climate is that no one else is going to maintain a comprehensive lifetime health record for you. Clinicians are required by law to document your medical encounters. We have not, however, evolved to a system that places the patient at the central point of the medical record when multiple providers are involved.

What happens when you move or switch providers? What happens when you change jobs and get new insurance? My personal medical record is effectively all over the country. I have lived in New Jersey, Vermont, and Texas, and I'm only about halfway done living. If I don't keep all the facts together, who will?

The importance of maintaining your own health record may not come to light during years of health, but having the record will prove invaluable over the course of your lifetime when your health status changes. As a child, I underwent abdominal surgery twice before the age of three. Had my parents maintained my health record, I would have found that information useful in my adult years.

Office Space

I have listed the key components needed for a comprehensive record. Storing this information in an organized fashion is paramount to your ability to communicate effectively and swiftly navigate your health care encounters. The data can be stored on paper in a manual file folder system or in combination with your home computer and a paper file system for the chart notes and diagnostic reports you receive from your providers.

The data are divided into two categories or folders, current information and historical information. Each folder should have five subsections:

1. Patient information and history (personal data that don't often change, including name, address, allergies, family history, etc.)

2. Insurance and reimbursement information, including explanation of benefits (EOBs)

3. Exam or encounter data

4. Legal documents

5. Contacts

I suggest you purchase a binder with dividers for each personal medical record you would like to create. If you intend to store this information on your computer, there will still be components of your record that will most likely need to be stored and organized on paper (unless you own a scanner, and therefore can store an image of the paper on your computer). Additionally, many health care providers are not ready to receive and send your data electronically, hence the necessity for paper.

There is no right or wrong way to store your information. What I have outlined below is a suggestion. I have done my best to optimize the model for a person using a computer with basic Word document and Excel spreadsheet layouts. If a computer is not available to you, simply copy the forms and create your record on paper in a binder or folder system. You can also download a free pdf of the forms at www.howtogetthehealthcareyouwant.com.

Create a binder for each patient's record you intend to maintain. You will need dividers labeled as listed below. Replace the word *patient* with the patient's name and clearly label the binder with the patient's name. Wherever I have bracketed a word, replace that word with the data requested between the brackets. For example, [Patient] would prompt you to enter the patient's name in that space—of course, leaving out the brackets.

Current: [Patient] Patient Information: Personal and Medical History

Current: [Patient] Insurance and Reimbursement

    Current: [Patient] Invoices and Explanation of Benefits

Current: [Patient] Exams and Encounters

Current: [Patient] Legal Documents

Current: [Patient] Contacts

History: [Patient] Patient Information: Personal Medical History

History: [Patient] Insurance and Reimbursement

    History: [Patient] Invoices and Explanation of Benefits

History: [Patient] Exams and Encounters

History: [Patient] Legal Documents

History: [Patient] Contacts

If you intend to use your computer, I suggest mirroring the binder and tab names on your computer as file folder names.

All of the forms outlined in this chapter have a footer to guide you as to where and how to file the form. In addition to where to store the data, each form has an effective date or last updated date labeling what period of time in the patient's life to which this information pertains. These dates are critical, as they will keep your records in chronological order.

As life progresses and your spouse changes jobs or you move, be sure to maintain your old data as well as update and keep your current data. In the paper model, you will do that by simply placing the newest paper at the beginning of each section. In the computer-based model you can store your documents by date so they can be sorted newest to oldest. A naming convention such as 20060108, representing January 8, 2006, would keep your electronic documents chronologically ordered.

Your Medical Record
Section 1: Patient Information

Create a patient information form each time the data change. Keep the new or current forms in your section titled Current. When data change on the current form, move the old "current" form to your section titled History in the folder named Patient Information and rename the form History. Include the following information in the patient information section.

Use a patient information form like the one in exhibit 6-1 to capture this data.

PATIENT ALLERGIES

Use this allergy listing as a guide to some common allergies. This list is by no means complete; add to it as is necessary for you.

Allergies Reactions to life-threatening food allergens could be immediate to less than one hour.

Avocados	Peanuts
Bananas	Sesame seeds
Chestnuts	Shellfish (shrimp, lobsters)
Chicken/Fowl	Soy
Eggs	Strawberries
Kiwi	Wheat
Milk	Tree nuts (almonds, pecans, walnuts, cashews)

Food Sensitivity These may not be life threatening, and reaction is typically more than one hour.

Aspartame (NutraSweet)	MSG
Cheese	Shellfish
Chocolate	Sulfite
Milk	Wine, beer

EXHIBIT 6-1 PATIENT INFORMATION FORM

PATIENT INFORMATION

Effective from: _____

Effective through: _____

Patient name: _____

Patient address: _____

Patient city: _____

Patient state: _____

Patient zip: _____

Patient home phone: _____

Patient cell phone: _____

Patient e-mail address: _____

Patient Social Security no. (optional): _____

Patient sex: _____

Patient primary language: _____

Patient height: _____

Patient weight: _____

Eye color: _____

Patient blood type: _____

Patient marital status: _____

Patient's number of children: _____

File: [Patient]/current/patient_info/ or when saving to history [Patient]/history/patient_info/[date]

Contact Allergy These may be life threatening for some people.

Band-Aids

Betadine

Cosmetics

Fragrances/perfumes

Large localized insect reactions (mosquitoes/spiders)

Latex/rubber

Nickel/jewelry

Plants (poison ivy, oak, sumac)

Topical antibiotics (Neosporin)

Airborne Allergens

Cockroach	Mold
Dog/cat	Smoke (from tobacco smoking)
Dust/dust mites	Tree pollen
Grass pollen	Weed pollen

Drug Allergy The reaction may be immediate or delayed.

Anticonvulsants	Ibuprofen, Aleve
Aspirin	IV contrast/iodine
Penicillin	Multiple antibiotic sensitivity
Beta-blocker medications	Multiple chemical sensitivity (MCS)
Cefaclor (Ceclor)	Sulfa drugs
Codeine/hydrocodone	ACE inhibitors (high blood pressure
Insulin	medication)

Possible Reactions to Allergens

Breathing problem	Itchy/watery eyes
Coughing	Nausea
Diarrhea	Rash
Dizziness	Runny nose
Fainting or passing out	Shock
Headache	Shortness of breath
Hives	Sneezing
Itching	Vomiting

You should complete an allergy form like the one in exhibit 6-2 for each allergy the patient has and store it in the Current folder in the Patient Information subsection Allergies. Should an allergy discontinue, then move that form to the folder called History in the Patient Information subsection under Allergies.

EXHIBIT 6-2 ALLERGY FORM

PATIENT INFORMATION ALLERGIES	Effective from: _____
	Effective through: _____

Patient name: _____

Allergen: _____

Reaction: _____

Date of onset: _____

Date of last episode: _____

Treatment method: _____

Doctor treating allergy: _____

File: [Patient]/current/patient_info/allergies/[Allergen]

PATIENT FAMILY HEALTH HISTORY

Use the medical history checklist in exhibit 6-3 to identify conditions, diagnoses, and procedures that apply to you and your family members. Use exhibit 6-4 to list surgical procedures. The lists by no means offer every possible condition, but they will serve as basic lists of common ailments and procedures. Add other conditions to the patient's history as they apply.

Create a medical history form like the one in exhibit 6-5 for all conditions, procedures, and surgeries. If the issues are currently part of your life, store the forms chronologically in the Current folder in the Patient Information subsection under Patient History. Note: You may not want to ever store your medical history in the history section of your record, as most physicians will be interested in your complete medical history. Storing this information in your Current folder will keep it accessible for all the physicians you encounter.

Use the family member information form in exhibit 6-6 as a guide to creating your family history. Most clinicians will want you to report clinical conditions for biological grandparents, parents, siblings (aunts/uncles), and the patient's siblings on both sides of your family.

EXHIBIT 6-3 MEDICAL HISTORY CHECKLIST

Abdominal pain (colic in infants)

Acne

ADHD/ADD

AIDS

Alcoholism

Alzheimer's disease

Anemia

Arthritis

Asthma

Athlete's foot

Autism

Bladder/kidney infections

Blocked tear duct

Blood clotting disorder

Breast lumps

Bronchitis

Bursitis

Canker sores

Carpal tunnel syndrome

Cataracts

Cellulites

Chickenpox

Chlamydia

Chronic constipation

Chronic obstructive pulmonary disease

Chronic pain

Colitis Crohn's disease

Colon polyps

Conjunctivitis (pink eye)

Corneal abrasions

Depression

Diabetes Type I

Diabetes Type II

Diarrhea

Dizziness

Drug dependency

Ear infections/hearing impairment

Eczema and psoriasis

Emphysema

Epilepsy

Eye problem

Fainting

Fibromyalgia

Gastritis

Gastro esophageal reflux disease (GERD)

Genital warts

Glaucoma

Gonorrhea

Gout

Hay Fever/sinus problems

Head lice

Hemodialysis

Hemorrhoids

Hepatitis

Hernia

Herpes

HIV positive

Hives

Hypoglycemia

Hypothyroidism

Impetigo

Incontinence

Infertility

Irritable bowel syndrome (IBS)

Jaundice

Kidney disease

Kidney failure

Limb pain

Liver problems

Low blood pressure

Lupus

Lyme disease

Measles

Meningitis

Mental health/psychiatric disorder

Migraine headache

Mononucleosis

Multiple Sclerosis

Mumps

Muscle disorder

Neck pain

Nose bleeds

Numbness

Open wounds

Osteoarthritis

Osteoporosis

Pain or pressure in chest

Palpitations

Paralysis

Parkinson's disease

Pelvic inflammatory disease

EXHIBIT 6-3 MEDICAL HISTORY CHECKLIST

Peptic ulcer disease

Periods of unconsciousness

Pertussis/whooping cough

Phlebitis

Pneumonia

Polio

Pulmonary embolism

Rash

Rectal bleeding

Rheumatic fever

Rheumatism

Ringworm

Rubella

Scabies

Scarlet fever

Scoliosis

Seizures/seizure disorder

Sexual dysfunction

Shingles

Shortness of breath (dyspnea)

Sickle cell

Sinus infection

Skin lesion

Smoking

Stomach or intestinal problems

Strep throat

Stroke

Swimmer's ear

Syphilis

Thyroid problems

Tonsillitis

Tuberculosis

Tumor

Upper respiratory infection

Urinary tract infections

Varicose veins

Warts

CANCER

Breast cancer

Colon/rectal cancer

Leukemia

Lung cancer

Non-Hodgkin's lymphoma

Ovarian cancer

Prostate cancer

Skin cancer

Urinary/bladder cancer

Uterine cancer

Other cancer

FEMALES

Abnormal PAP

Bleeding problems

Breast mass or cyst

Contraceptions

Cyst or abscess of vulva

Discomfort with sex

Endometriosis

Fibroids

Irregular periods

Menopause

Miscarriage

Nipple discharge

Ovarian cysts

Postmenopausal bleeding

Postpartum depression

Pregnancy

Toxemia

Tubal pregnancy

CHILDREN

Birthmarks

Cradle cramp

Croup

Hand, foot, and mouth disease

Mental retardation

Pinworms

Roseola (baby measles)

MALES

Prostate problems

EXHIBIT 6-4 SURGERIES AND PROCEDURES

Abdominal surgery	CT scan	Mammogram
Abortion	Cystoscopy	Mastectomy
Angiogram	Dialysis	MRI
Angioplasty	Dilation & curettage (D&C)	Myelogram
Ankle/leg fracture repair	Electrocardiogram (EKG)	Ophorectomy
Appendectomy	Episiotomy	Pacemaker
Arterial line placement	Fusions (e.g., lumbar)	PET scan
Artificial insemination	Gall bladder removal (cholecsystectomy)	Prostatectomy
Aspiration of breast cyst	Gastroscopy	Pulmonary artery catheter placement
Back surgery	Glaucoma surgery	Radial keratotomy (RK)
Bladder repair	Heart bypass surgery	Radiation treatment
Blood transfusion	Heart valve replacement	Radiograph
Bone scan	Hemorrhoid surgery	Shoulder surgery
Cardiac catheterization	Hernia repair	Sigmoidoscopy
Carpal tunnel surgery	Hip replacement	Spinal tap/lumbar puncture
Cataract surgery	Hysterectomy	Splenectomy
Cesarean section	In-vitro fertilization (IVF)	Stress test
Chemotherapy	Joint aspiration	Thyroidectomy
Chest tube placement	Knee replacement	Tonsillectomy
Circumcision	Knee surgery	Tracheostomy
Colonoscopy	Laminectomy	Transuretheral prostate surgery
Colorectal resection	Laparoscopy	Tubal ligation (female sterilization)
Colposcopy	Laparotomy	
Coronary artery bypass grafting (CABG)	LASIK	Ultrasound
Cosmetic surgery	LEEP	Vasectomy (male sterilization)
Craniotomy	Lumpectomy	

EXHIBIT 6-5 MEDICAL HISTORY FORM

PATIENT INFORMATION MEDICAL HISTORY   Effective from: _____

                                          Effective through: _____

Patient name: _____

Condition: _____

Is this condition active or resolved?   _____

Doctor treating this condition: _____

Date of onset: _____

Date of diagnosis: _____

Date of treatment: _____

Method of treatment: _____

Medication: _____

Diet: _____

Exercise: _____

Hospitalization: _____

Surgery: _____

Date of surgery: _____

Affected body area: _____

Outcome: _____

Doctor who performed the
surgery or procedure: _____

Therapy: _____

Other: _____

Date of resolution: _____

File: [Patient]/current/patient_info/med_history/[date of condition]

The second question in exhibit 6-6 asks for the relationship this family member has to the patient. Remember to be specific in identifying how this relative is connected (i.e., what side of the family). If the person is your mother's sister, then indicate *maternal aunt*. If the person is your father's father, then indicate *paternal grandfather*.

EXHIBIT 6-6 FAMILY MEDICAL HISTORY

FAMILY MEMBER INFORMATION
MEDICAL HISTORY

Effective from: _____

Effective through: _____

Family member name: _____

Family member relation to patient: _____

Patient name: _____

Is this family member living? _____

If this family member is deceased, cause of death? _____

Condition: _____

Is this condition active or resolved? _____

Date of onset: _____

Date of treatment: _____

Method of treatment: _____

Medication: _____

Hospitalization: _____

Surgery: _____

Date of surgery: _____

Affected body area: _____

Outcome: _____

Doctor who performed the surgery or procedure: _____

File: [Patient]/current/patient_info/[family member]/med_history/[condition/[date of condition]

COMMON IMMUNIZATIONS

Create an immunization form for each immunization the patient has received. If you have your immunization record, you can simply copy it and add it to your personal medical record. Include the dates for all immunizations. This information should be stored in [Patient]/current/patient_info/ medical_history/immunizations. The following are possible immunizations. Some are required by the school systems, some are recommended, and others are only needed under specific circumstances.

Anthrax	Meningococcal vaccine
Chickenpox (Varicella or VZV)	Mumps
Cholera	Pertussis/whooping cough
Diphtheria	Plague
Haemophilus influenza type b (Hib)	Pneumococcal conjugate vaccine (PCV7 or PCV)
Hepatitis A (Hep A)	Polio (IPV)
Hepatitis B (Hep B)	Rabies
Immune serum	Diphtheria/tetanus/pertussis
Influenza	Measles/mumps/rubella (MMR)
Japanese encephalitis	Tetanus and diphtheria booster (Td)
Lyme disease	Other:_____

Use this information to fill out an immunization chart, such as exhibit 6-7.

MEDICATIONS

The medications form like the one in exhibit 6-8 tracks current and historic medications. Complete one for every medication. Store current medications in [Patient]/current/patient_info/medical_history/medications/[date]. If you are no longer using a medication, move the form to [Patient]/history/ patient_info/medical_history/medications/[date].

EXHIBIT 6-7 RECORD OF IMMUNIZATIONS

PATIENT IMMUNIZATIONS   Last updated: _____

Patient name: _____

    Immunization: _____

    Date given: _____

    Doctor: _____

    Immunization: _____

    Date given: _____

    Doctor: _____

    Immunization: _____

    Date given: _____

    Doctor: _____

    Immunization: _____

    Date given: _____

    Doctor: _____

File: [Patient]/current/patient_info/medical_history/immunizations

NUTRITION SUPPORT

If you've been placed on a special diet, use a nutrition form like exhibit 6-9 to indicate your diet and any food restrictions you have. Store this form in [Patient]/current/patient_info/medical_history/Nutrition or if you are no longer required to be on this diet store the form in [Patient]/history/ patient_info/medical_history/nutrition/[date]. The following list contains common nutritional supplements.

Common Pediatric Nutrition	Common Adult Nutrition
Advera	Allmentum
ELeCare	Ensure
Glucerna	Juven
Nepro	Pedialyte
Rehydrate	Similac NeoSure

EXHIBIT 6-8 MEDICATIONS

PATIENT MEDICATIONS   Last updated: _____

Patient name: _____

Medication: _____

Medication start date: _____

Medication end date: _____

Condition being treated: _____

Medication strength (e.g., 800 mg):   _____

Medication form (e.g., tablet):   _____

Medication frequency
(e.g., 3 times per day):   _____

Medication duration (e.g., 10 days):   _____

Medication directions: _____

Doctor prescribing this medication: _____

Date of prescription: _____

Pharmacy name and phone number: _____

Prescription number: _____

File: [Patient]/current/patient_info/medical_history/medications/[date]

EXHIBIT 6-9 DIET AND NUTRITION PLAN

PATIENT NUTRITION   Last updated: _____

Patient name: _____

Diet plan: _____

Dietary restrictions: _____

Dietary supplements: _____

File: [Patient]/current/patient_info/medical_history/Nutrition/[date]

Your Medical Record Section 2: Insurance and Financial Information

In clinical settings, health-related documentation is not typically mixed with your insurance or financial information. You, however, still need to monitor your insurance company and providers to ensure your bills and claims are paid appropriately. Another benefit to storing the information is the annual budgeting process will be more efficient because you will have the historic health-related costs organized. You will be able to easily trend your expenditures. Lastly, in case you may be wondering why you should keep insurance information with your personal medical history, I ask, have you ever gotten a bill from a provider two years after the date of service and you have no recollection of what insurance you had at the time? If not, consider yourself lucky, as it's been known to happen. Keep your old insurance cards and tape them to your coverage page in the history section of your personal health record.

Each time you move, you change jobs, or your employer changes insurance plans, you should update your insurance and financial information and then store the old information in history. Current information is stored in [Patient]/current/Insurance_info and history is stored in [Patient]/history/Insurance_info/[date]. Use a form like exhibit 6-10 to track your information.

Explanation of Benefits

Keep all copies of explanation of benefits (EOBs), or remittance advice, from your insurance company for at least three years. If you ever receive a rogue bill from a provider two-and-a-half years after the service was performed, you can quickly and easily research whether your insurance paid the claim or whether the claim was even filed, and if you paid a deductible or coinsurance. Another suggestion is to notate your check number on the EOB so it will be easy to find your check in the event you need to prove you paid for the service. [Patient]/history/Insurance_info/EOBs/[date] is a subsection of [Patient]/history/Insurance_info/[date].

EXHIBIT 6-10 INSURANCE AND EMPLOYER INFORMATION

INSURANCE AND EMPLOYER INFORMATION

Effective from: _____

Effective through: _____

Patient name: _____

Patient address: _____

Patient city, state, zip: _____

Patient home phone: _____

Patient cell phone: _____

Patient e-mail address: _____

Patient Social Security no. (optional): _____

Patient sex: _____

Patient primary language: _____

Guarantor name: _____

Guarantor address: _____

Guarantor city, state, zip: _____

Guarantor home phone: _____

Guarantor cell phone: _____

Guarantor e-mail address: _____

Guarantor Social Security no.: (opt.) _____

Primary insurance company name: _____

Primary insurance company claims address: _____

Primary insurance company claims address, city, state, and zip: _____

Primary insurance company claims phone number: _____

Primary insurance company claims fax number: _____

Primary insurance subscriber name: _____

Primary insurance subscriber address: _____

Primary insurance subscriber city, state, zip: _____

Primary insurance subscriber telephone: _____

Primary insurance subscriber employer name: _____

Primary insurance subscriber employer address: _____

Primary insurance subscriber employer city, state, and zip: _____

Patient relationship to subscriber: _____

Secondary insurance company name: _____

Secondary insurance company claims address: _____

Secondary insurance company claims address, city, state, and zip: _____

Secondary insurance company claims phone number: _____

Secondary insurance company claims fax number: _____

Secondary insurance subscriber name: _____

Secondary insurance subscriber address: _____

Secondary insurance subscriber city, state, zip; _____

Secondary insurance subscriber telephone: _____

Secondary insurance subscriber employer name: _____

Secondary insurance subscriber employer address: _____

Secondary insurance subscriber employer city, state, and zip: _____

Patient relationship to secondary subscriber: _____

Tertiary insurance company name: _____

Tertiary insurance company claims address: _____

Tertiary insurance company claims address, city, state, and zip: _____

Tertiary insurance company claims
phone number: _____

Tertiary insurance company claims
fax number: _____

Tertiary insurance subscriber name: _____

Tertiary insurance subscriber
address: _____

Tertiary insurance subscriber city,
state, zip: _____

Tertiary insurance subscriber
telephone: _____

Tertiary insurance subscriber
employer name: _____

Tertiary insurance subscriber
employer address: _____

Tertiary insurance subscriber
employer city, state, and zip: _____

Patient relationship to tertiary
subscriber: _____

Employer information: _____

Patient employer name: _____

Patient employer address: _____

Patient employer city, state, zip: _____

Patient employer phone: _____

Guarantor employer name: _____

Guarantor employer address: _____

Guarantor employer city, state, zip: _____

Guarantor employer phone: _____

File: [Patient]/Insurance_info/current

Note: provide a copy of the front and back of your current insurance card.

Your Medical Record
Section 3: Exams and Encounters

This section of your medical record will be a blend of your own record keeping and your clinician's record keeping. I have reviewed much of what you want to think about and monitor as you experience health care providers and facilities in previous chapters. For this section of your health record, I will tie all of those pieces together for you. Exhibit 6-11 provides a good overview.

EXHIBIT 6-11 STANDARD CARE EXPECTATIONS AND PERSONAL PREFERENCES

PERSONAL PREFERENCES

Patient: _____

Date: _____

1. Care means _____ to me.
2. I am seeking care because _____.
3. I believe _____ will cure me.
4. List life stressors that may be contributing to this illness: (for example)

My job	My parent
My marriage	Loss of loved one
My divorce	Loss of job
My child	Abusive relationship
My home	Drug or alcohol abuse

5. To what level or degree do I want to participate in the decision-making process of my care?
6. I want a male/female doctor.
7. I care/don't care about the physician's primary language. I want that language to be _____.
8. I want my doctor to have been in practice _____ years.
9. I need this doctor to integrate with a team of doctors already working on my issue. (List the team members.)
10. I will bring the care team's contact sheet with me to this visit.
11. I need to communicate my expectation that the team communicate well among itself.
12. I expect my clinician to be an M.D., PA, Intern, etc. (See chapter 4 definitions.)

ACCESS

1. I expect to be seen in _____ hours/days/weeks/months.

2. I expect the appointment booking encounter to take less than _____ minutes/hours/days/ months.

3. I expect to wait no more than _____ minutes/hours/days/weeks for my health care service.

4. I expect to describe my symptoms/situations or tell my story to no more than _____ person(s). I have prepared a health record for this illness/exam and will share it with my doctor in a written format.

5. I expect to provide my personal and insurance information to no more than ____ person(s). I will bring my personal medical and family history in written form to all appointments when I am meeting with a new doctor.

6. I expect to pay _____ dollars for this service.

7. On a scale of zero to ten, my tolerance for redundancies and inefficiencies is ___ (zero being not at all tolerant and ten being extremely tolerant).

8. On a scale of zero to ten, my tolerance for timeliness is___ (zero being not at all tolerant and ten being extremely tolerant).

9. I expect to spend _____ hours/days/weeks/months/lifetime healing this health issue OR I will ask my doctor how long I should expect to spend healing this issue.

STANDARD CARE QUESTIONS

1. Do I really need the care they are proposing?

2. Do I really need the medications they are prescribing?

3. Will this treatment plan enhance my quality of life and wellness?

4. Years in practice?

5. Medical school graduate of _____

6. Internship performed at _____

7. Undergraduate degree in _____ from _____

8. Why did you become a _____ doctor?

9. How do you prepare for exams or procedures?

10. Will you read chart notes and documentation other doctors send to you before I arrive for my appointments?

11. What was the most exciting thing you learned recently that pertains to your career as a _____ doctor?

12. If we mutually agree that this relationship is a match, will you be committed to my care until I am well (or for my lifetime, in the case of a primary or family care situation) _____?

13. Have you ever had your hospital privileges revoked? If yes, where and why?

14. How would you feel if I were to need a second or third opinion pertaining to my health? How would you facilitate my request?

15. Considering I (the patient) track my medical history and will require my doctor(s) to read my history and share their charting with me, how did this doctor respond when I explained that? How will he/she share my chart notes with me? Via fax? USPS? Secure e-mail? Is the provider willing to share a photocopy of my record each day I am seen or remain in the hospital?

16. Understanding we are all humans and humans make mistakes, can you in general terms describe a mistake you made and what you did to rectify the situation?
17. Can you have three patients with my similar health status contact me as references?
18. Who will call me with test results? Will it be you, the doctor, or do you delegate that to a nurse?
19. Can I request that you call me with the results?
20. Will you mail, or fax my results to me?
21. How quickly will I get my results from you?
22. If I am in the hospital are you willing to book an appointment (or perform your rounds) at a mutually agreed upon time (e.g., not 5:45 a.m.) so that I can have my advocate present?

Add you own questions.

COMMUNICATION AND REACTIONS

1. Was my initial reaction to this person a perception of a caring individual?
2. Did the person introduce himself or herself in a comfortable, approachable confident way?
3. How did the conversation flow?
4. Was the person a good listener?
5. Did he/she maintain good eye contact?
6. Did I understand what the person was saying?
7. Did the person ask well-rounded questions?
8. Did the questions expand beyond the scope of the one section of my body that is ailing? In a primary care situation, did the questions include my entire body, my emotional state, my family, and my life?
9. Did I leave feeling comfortable with this person?
10. Could I trust this person with my life?
11. Is there some sort of bond with this person?
12. Do I feel safe?
13. Is the communication easy and flowing? If I didn't understand something, did the person take the time to ensure that I understood?
14. Can this doctor comply with most or all of my standard expectations?
15. What does my intuition (or gut) tell me about this person?
16. Did this person do what he or she said they were going to do?

INSURANCE AND FINANCE

1. Is this doctor part of my insurance network?
2. Does this doctor plan to remain part of my insurance network? (If this doctor changes or cancels contracts with insurance companies on a regular basis, then you will either need to incur greater cost to continue care with this provider or need to seek care from another provider.)
3. Does this doctor have organized business practices?
4. What are the billing and collections policies?

File: [Patient]/current/clinical_encounters/expectations

PREVISIT NOTES

Certainly, there are instances when you cannot prepare for a health care–related visit. You can, however use the previsit notes section to recollect your experience when an urgent matter has required the need of medical care and track your thoughts, questions, feelings, etc., after the fact. Use the SOAP method described in chapter 2 and outlined below, and make out a chart like exhibit 6-12.

- Subjective, or what is important and relevant positive and negative information. This information could be your history or a description of what is currently going on with your body and life. In other words, tell your story.
- Objective, or important findings. This includes data such as test results or physical statistics.
- Assessment, a priority listing of what you believe is wrong—in other words, your diagnosis. What do you feel needs attention? How is your life affected and what are your priorities?
- Plan, what's next? What are your questions, concerns, and criticisms? What is your ideal treatment path? How does this problem get resolved.[5]

CREATING AN ANXIETY GRAPH

Create your anxiety graph for the encounter. Label the x-axis with your experiences, then plot your emotion or anxiety levels during those experiences for this encounter. Do your best to separate your anxiety associated with your care from the anxiety associated from the actual illness. Focus on how your anxiety changes as it relates to the care you are receiving. Refer to chapter 3 to see how to chart your anxiety, using a graph like the one in exhibit 6-13.

EXHIBIT 6-12 SOAP NOTES

PREVISIT SOAP NOTES   Patient: _____

                                             Date: _____

Provider: _____

Condition or chief complaint: _____

S: What do I need to tell the caregiver(s) (give them positive and negative thoughts,
   feelings, signs, and symptoms). Tell the story.

_____

_____

O: What are the important and relevant physical changes since your last visit? Bring your
   lab test results.

_____

_____

A: What do you believe is wrong? What do you feel needs attention? How is your life
   affected, and what are your priorities?

_____

_____

P: What is your plan? What are your questions, concerns, and criticisms? What is your
   ideal treatment path? How does this problem get resolved?

_____

_____

My Standard Care Questions are: [copy from your preferences where applicable]

File: [Patient]/current/clinical_encounters/previsit_questions/[provider]/[visit date]

TAKING NOTES

Create a section for visit notes and store the notes you take or the notes
your advocate takes. Exhibit 6-14 is an example.

EXHIBIT 6-13 ANXIETY LEVEL GRAPH

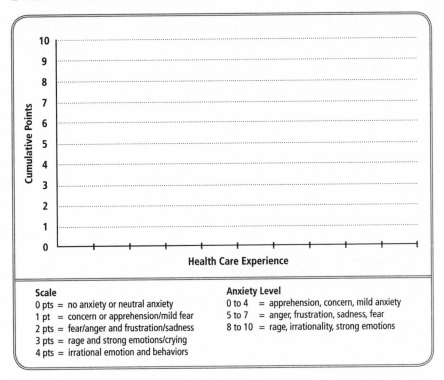

Scale
0 pts = no anxiety or neutral anxiety
1 pt = concern or apprehension/mild fear
2 pts = fear/anger and frustration/sadness
3 pts = rage and strong emotions/crying
4 pts = irrational emotion and behaviors

Anxiety Level
0 to 4   = apprehension, concern, mild anxiety
5 to 7   = anger, frustration, sadness, fear
8 to 10 = rage, irrationality, strong emotions

EXHIBIT 6-14 ENCOUNTER NOTES

ENCOUNTER NOTES

Patient: _____

Date: _____

Provider: _____

Reason for encounter: _____

Notes: .   _____

_____

_____

_____

_____

File: [Patient]/current/clinical_encounters/notes/[provider]/[visit date]

RECORD KEEPING

The last section of your clinical encounters is all the data you receive from your clinicians. Make the follow sections per condition or issue and store the information in chronological order:

- Chart notes stored by provider
- Diagnostic exam results
  - Lab
  - X-ray

Your Medical Record
Section 4: Legal Documents

MEDICAL POWER OF ATTORNEY

The purpose of a medical power of attorney is to delegate or appoint someone to make care decisions for the patient. This type of document is necessary when the patient is unable to communicate his or her treatment preferences and choices.

The patient at the time of signing the document must be a competent adult. Execution of the form denotes a person (the patient's agent) who the patient trusts to make health care decisions on his or her behalf. The power of attorney takes effect when it is signed by all parties and remains in effect indefinitely, unless the document specifies a termination date. The agent can only make decisions on behalf of the patient if the patient's attending physician certifies in writing that the patient is incompetent. The agent cannot make a health care decision if the patient objects to that decision.

Considering there is a chance during the course of your lifetime that you may become seriously injured, ill, or unable to make decisions regarding health care, it would be helpful to have someone who knows your values and can act on your behalf.

Medical power of attorney forms can be obtained from most large health care providers or your state medical society. The forms are driven by state law, so you will need to get a version that pertains to your state.

LIVING WILL

A living will is a legal document in which you state the type of care you want or don't want under certain circumstances.

DO NOT RESUSCITATE (DNR) ORDER

A DNR order allows patients, for example, to direct health care providers outside the hospital setting to withhold or withdraw specific life-sustaining treatments in the event of respiratory or cardiac arrest (this varies by state). The DNR order is created at the patient's request and cannot be made a requirement of care for any reason (including issuance of insurance or a provision of care).

If the patient is a minor the DNR order can only be executed when the minor has been diagnosed by a physician as suffering from a terminal or irreversible condition.

Check your state department of health for guidelines and access to the form and state laws most appropriate for you.

ORGAN DONOR

I would suggest making your family aware that you wish to donate organs as a first step. Call the Living Bank at 800-528-2971. It serves as an organ donation education center and national organ registry. Request an organ donor form, complete the form, and return it to the Living Bank.

Many states offer the ability to sign up for organ donation with your driver's license renewal, and there is no harm to your driver's license indicating you are an organ donor in addition to your organ donation card.

Store your legal documents in the Current section of your medical record. Use a basic cover sheet, as in exhibit 6-15, to identify what documents you have and when they were signed.

EXHIBIT 6-15 COVER SHEET

Medical power of attorney	Yes	No
Date signed:		
Document location:		
Living will	Yes	No
Date signed:		
Document location:		
Do not resuscitate order (DNR)	Yes	No
Date signed:		
Document location:		
Organ donor	Yes	No
Date signed:		
Document location:		

Your Medical Record
Section 5: Contacts

You may choose to store your contacts in Outlook or a Rolodex file. I recommend you keep past contacts in the History folder just in case you need them in the future. If you want to maintain consistency with the other forms, the following section outlines a structure for the contacts you should maintain. Exhibit 6-16 is an example of a contact sheet for doctors and clinicians who might be current or past providers.

Exhibit 6-17 is the area to store your pharmacy contact information. Exhibit 6-18 is an example of a contact sheet containing important health insurance information. You also might want employer contact information, as shown in exhibit 6-19; emergency contact information, shown in exhibit 6-20; and caregiver contact information, shown in exhibit 6-21. Finally, it is good to have a facilities contact sheet, as shown in exhibit 6-22.

EXHIBIT 6-16 CLINICIAN CONTACTS

CLINICIAN CONTACTS   Last updated: _____

Last name: _____

First name: _____

Phone number: _____

Fax: _____

Specialty: _____

Address: _____

Address: _____

City: _____

State: _____

Zip: _____

File:[Patient]/current/contacts/doctors/[clinician last name]

EXHIBIT 6-17 PHARMACY

PHARMACY CONTACTS   Last updated: _____

Pharmacy: _____

Phone number: _____

Fax: _____

Address: _____

Address: _____

City: _____

State: _____

Zip: _____

File: [Patient]/current/contacts/pharmacy/[pharmacy name]

EXHIBIT 6-18 HEALTH INSURANCE CONTACTS

CONTACTS FOR INSURANCE COMPANIES   Effective from: _____

Effective through: _____

Primary insurance company name: _____

   Customer service phone number: _____

   Customer service fax: _____

   Customer service address: _____

   Customer service address: _____

   Customer service city, state, & zip: _____

   Claims phone number: _____

   Claims fax number: _____

   Claims address: _____

   Claims address: _____

   Claims city, state, & zip: _____

   Company Web address: _____

   Company e-mail address: _____

Secondary insurance company name: _____

   Customer service phone number: _____

   Customer service fax: _____

   Customer service address: _____

   Customer service address: _____

   Customer service city, state, & zip: _____

   Claims phone number: _____

   Claims fax number: _____

   Claims address: _____

   Claims address: _____

   Claims city, state, & zip: _____

   Insurance company Web address: _____

   Insurance company e-mail address: _____

Tertiary insurance company name: _____

   Customer service phone number: _____

   Customer service fax: _____

Customer service address: _____

Customer service address: _____

Customer service address: _____

Customer service city, state, & zip: _____

Claims phone number: _____

Claims fax number: _____

Claims address: _____

Claims address: _____

Claims city, state, & zip: _____

Insurance company Web address: _____

Insurance company e-mail address: _____

File: [Patient]/current/contacts/ins_Info/[Insurance_Co_name]

EXHIBIT 6-19 EMPLOYER CONTACT INFORMATION

EMPLOYER CONTACT INFORMATION   Effective from: _____

Effective through: _____

Employer name: _____

Employer for whom? _____

Employer address: _____

Employer address: _____

Customer service address: _____

Employer city, state, & zip: _____

Employer phone: _____

Employer fax: _____

Employer human resource
representative: _____

Employer human resource phone: _____

Employer e-mail: _____

Employer Web address: _____

File: [Patient]/current/contacts/employer/[employer_name]

EXHIBIT 6-20 EMERGENCY CONTACT INFORMATION

EMERGENCY CONTACT INFORMATION

Effective from: _____

Effective through: _____

Emergency contact name: _____

Emergency contact phone: _____

Emergency contact cell phone: _____

Emergency contact work phone: _____

Emergency contact address: _____

Emergency contact address: _____

Emergency contact city, state, & zip: _____

Emergency contact fax: _____

File: [Patient]/current/contacts/emergency/[contact last name]

EXHIBIT 6-21 CAREGIVER CONTACT INFORMATION

CAREGIVER CONTACTS

Effective from: _____

Effective through: _____

Caregiver contact name: _____

Caregiver role: _____

Relationship to the guarantor: _____

Caregiver contact phone: _____

Caregiver cell phone: _____

Caregiver work phone: _____

Caregiver address: _____

Caregiver city, state, & zip: _____

Caregiver fax: _____

Caregiver schedule: _____

Caregiver company: _____

Caregiver company phone: _____

Caregiver company address: _____

Caregiver company address: _____

Caregiver company city, state, & zip: _____

Caregiver company fax: _____

File: [Patient]/current/contacts/care_giver/[caregiver last name]

EXHIBIT 6-22 FACILITIES CONTACTS

FACILITIES CONTACTS   Last updated: _____

Facility or hospital name: _____

Phone number: _____

Fax: _____

Address: _____

Address: _____

City: _____

State: _____

Zip: _____

Facility Web address: _____

Facility e-mail address: _____

File: [Patient]/current/contacts/facilities/[facility name]

Bringing It All Together

Use all the data stored in your Current folder when interacting with providers. Effectively, you should be able to simply copy all your forms and
hand a new provider your entire health record, current personal information, and current insurance and employer information in one fell swoop.
That step gets you out of completing redundant paperwork and telling
your story to five different people.

Remember those friendly front desk staff members from chapter 3?
They are going to tell you, "You *have* to fill out our forms." You may need to
sign their form committing to pay, indicating you have received and agree
with their privacy form, or that you consent to treatment, but they can take
the comprehensive data you are diligently providing in your format and figure it all out from there. Be ready for resistance. You might want to separate
your information into two packets, one for business-related issues and one
for clinical issues. Be sure to record in your encounter notes exactly who you
provided your information to in the event the information is lost.

Simply hand your personal and insurance information packet over to the front desk and the other packet to the physician. The more organized you are, the more respect you should command from people who do care and are truly professionals, with your health at the center of their mission. Ask for copies of all the forms you do sign and store them with your encounter information.

As you experience the interaction with staff and the providers, write down your feelings and questions and answers, and keep those notes in the Encounter section of your medical record in the event you need to revisit them in the future. Use all of this data to communicate the good, and the bad, to your providers and facilities.

When you have complex care needs, meaning you are traveling for care or you need a team of individuals to work together so your care is optimized, take your Current and History sections of your medical record and copy the pertinent portions for *all* the caregivers involved. Be sure to include you contacts so that each caregiver has the means to contact the others when necessary. In other words, make packets of information for each member of the team and date and label the packet (e.g., 5/15/06 v.3) so everyone can stay on the same page.

If you are receiving care in a city different from where you live and you need the caregivers in the foreign city to communicate with your local providers, schedule a conference call to your local provider the next time you are with the provider in the far-away locale. That way, you are present for the conversation and are aware the introduction did take place.

7

Resources

- - - - - - - - - - - - - - - - -

American Board of Medical Specialties

American Board of Medical Specialties
1007 Church Street, Suite 404 | Evanston, IL 60201-5913
Phone Verification (866) ASK-ABMS
(847) 491-9091 | Fax: (847) 328-3596
www.abms.org

The purpose of the American Board of Medical Specialties is to provide assurance to the public that a certified medical specialist has successfully completed and approved an educational program and an evaluation, including an examination process designed to assess the knowledge, experience, and skills requisite to the provisions of high-quality patient care in the specialty the physician has chosen to practice.

Which Medical Specialist Is for You?

The following content can be found on www.abms.org, the American Board of Medical Specialties® website. The descriptions may help you determine what kind of doctor your need. See exhibit 7-1 for addresses and websites related to each specialty.

EXHIBIT 7-1 RESOURCE LIST FOR ABMS SPECIALISTS

Allergy & Immunology
111 S. Independence
Mall East, Ste. 701
Philadelphia, PA 19106-3699
(215) 592-9466
www.abai.org

Anesthesiology
4101 Lake Boone Trail, Ste. 510
Raleigh, NC 27607-7506
(919) 881-2570
www.theaba.org

Colon & Rectal Surgery
20600 Eureka Road, Ste. 600
Taylor, MI 48180
(734) 282-9400
www.abcrs.org

Dermatology
Henry Ford Health System
1 Ford Place
Detroit, MI 48202-3450
(313) 874-1088
www.abderm.org

Emergency Medicine
3000 Coolidge Road
East Lansing, MI 48823-6319
(517) 332-4800
www.abem.org

Family Medicine
2228 Young Drive
Lexington, KY 40505-4294
(859) 269-5626
www.theabfm.org

Internal Medicine
510 Walnut Street, Ste. 1700
Philadelphia, PA 19106-3699
(215) 446-3500
www.abim.org

Medical Genetics
9650 Rockville Pike
Bethesda, MD 20814-3998
(301) 634-7316
www.abmg.org

Neurological Surgery
6550 Fannin Street, Ste. 2139
Houston, TX 77030-2701
(713) 441-6015
www.abns.org

Nuclear Medicine
4555 Forest Park Blvd., Ste. 119
St. Louis, MO 63108
(314) 367-2225
www.abnm.org

Obstetrics & Gynecology
2915 Vine Street, Ste. 300
Dallas, TX 75204
(214) 871-1619
www.abog.org

Ophthalmology
111 Presidential Blvd, Ste. 241
Bala Cynwyd, PA 19004-1075
(610) 664-1175
www.abop.org

Orthopaedic Surgery
400 Silver Cedar Court
Chapel Hill, NC 27514
(919) 929-7103
www.abos.org

Otolaryngology
5615 Kirby Drive, Ste. 600
Houston, TX 77005
(713) 850-0399
www.aboto.org

Pathology
P.O. Box 25915
Tampa, FL 33622-5915
(813) 286-2444
www.abpath.org

Pediatrics
111 Silver Cedar Court
Chapel Hill, NC 27514-1651
(919) 929-0461
www.abp.org

Physical Medicine & Rehabilitation
3015 Allegro Park Lane SW
Rochester, MN 55902-4139
(507) 282-1776
www.abpmr.org

Plastic Surgery
Seven Penn Center, Ste. 400
1635 Market Street
Philadelphia, PA 19103-2204
(215) 587-9322
www.abplsurg.org

Preventive Medicine
330 South Wells St., Ste. 1018
Chicago, IL 60606-7106
(312) 939-2276
www.abprevmed.org

Psychiatry & Neurology
500 Lake Cook Road, Ste. 335
Deerfield, IL 60015-5249
(847) 945-7900
www.abpn.org

Radiology
5441 East Williams Blvd., Ste. 200
Tucson, AZ 85711
(520) 790-2900
www.theabr.org

Surgery
1617 John F. Kennedy Blvd.,
Ste. 860
Philadelphia, PA 19103-1847
(215) 568-4000
www.absurgery.org

Thoracic Surgery
633 N. St. Clair St., Ste. 2320
Chicago, IL 60611
(312) 202-5900
www.abts.org

Urology
2216 Ivy Road, Ste. 210
Charlottesville, VA 22903
(434) 979-0059
www.abu.org

ABMS ASSOCIATE MEMBERS

Accreditation Council for
Graduate Medical Education
515 North State Street, Ste. 2000
Chicago, IL 60610-4322
(312) 755-5000
www.acgme.org

Accreditation Council for
Continuing Medical Education
515 N. State Street, Ste. 2150
Chicago, IL 60610
(312) 755-7401
www.accme.org

American Hospital Association
One North Franklin
Chicago, IL 60606-3421
(312) 422-3000
www.aha.org

American Medical Association
515 N. State St.
Chicago, IL 60610
(800) 621-8335
www.ama-assn.org

Association of American Medical
Colleges
2450 N Street, NW
Washington, DC 20037-1126
(202) 828-0400
www.aamc.org

Council of Medical Specialty
Societies
51 Sherwood Terrace, Ste. M
Lake Bluff, IL 60044-2232
(847) 295-3456
www.cmss.org

Educational Commission for
Foreign Medical Graduates
3624 Market Street
Philadelphia, PA 19104-2685
(215) 386-5900
www.ecfmg.org

Federation of State Medical
Boards
400 Fuller Wiser Road, Ste. 300
Euless, TX 76039-3855
(817) 868-4000
www.fsmb.org

National Board of Medical
Examiners
3750 Market Street
Philadelphia, PA 19104-3102
(215) 590-9500
www.nbme.org

ALLERGY AND IMMUNOLOGY

An allergist-immunologist is trained in evaluation, physical and laboratory diagnosis, and management of disorders involving the immune system. Selected examples of such conditions include asthma, anaphylaxis, rhinitis, eczema, and adverse reactions to drugs, foods, and insect stings, as well as immune deficiency diseases (both acquired and congenital), defects in host defense, and problems related to autoimmune disease, organ transplantation, or malignancies of the immune system. As our understanding of the immune system develops, the scope of this specialty is widening.

Training Required: prior certification in internal medicine or pediatrics; two years in allergy/immunology

Subspecialty
- *Clinical and laboratory immunology* This subspecialist utilizes various laboratory procedures to diagnose and treat disorders characterized by defective responses of the body's immune system. These results are used for patient management.

ANESTHESIOLOGY

An anesthesiologist is trained to provide pain relief and maintenance, or restoration of a stable condition during and immediately following an operation, an obstetric procedure, or diagnostic procedure. The anesthesiologist assesses the risk of the patient undergoing surgery and optimizes the patient's condition prior to, during, and after surgery. In addition to these management responsibilities, the anesthesiologist provides medical management and consultation in pain management and critical care medicine. Anesthesiologists diagnose and treat acute, long-standing, and cancer pain problems; diagnose and treat patients with critical illnesses or severe injuries; direct resuscitation in the care of patients with cardiac or respiratory emergencies, including the need to artificial ventilations; and supervise postanesthesia recovery.

Training Required: four years

Subspecialties
- *Critical care medicine* The anesthesiologist who specializes in critical care medicine diagnosis treats and supports patients with multiple organ dysfunction. This specialist may have administrative responsibilities for intensive care units and may also facilitate and coordinate patient care among the primary physician, the critical care staff, and other specialties.

- *Pain management* The anesthesiologist provides a high level of care, either as a primary physician or consultant, for patients experiencing problems with acute, chronic and/or cancer pain in both hospital and ambulatory settings. Patient care needs may also be coordinated with other specialists.

COLON AND RECTAL SURGERY

A colon and rectal surgeon is trained to diagnose and treat various diseases of the intestinal tract, colon, rectum, anal canal, and perianal area by medical and surgical means. This specialist also deals with other organs and tissues (such as the liver, urinary, and female reproductive system) involved with primary intestinal disease.

Colon and rectal surgeons have the expertise to diagnose and manage anorectal conditions such as hemorrhoids, fissures (painful tears in the anal lining), abscesses, and fistulae (infections located around the anus and rectum). They also treat problems of the intestines and colon, and perform endoscopic procedures to evaluate and treat problems such as cancer, polyps (precancerous growths), and inflammatory conditions.

Training required: six years

DERMATOLOGY

A dermatologist is trained to diagnose and treat pediatric and adult patients with benign and malignant disorders of the skin, mouth, external genitalia, hair and nails, as wells as a number of sexually transmitted diseases. The dermatologist has had additional training and experience in the diagnosis and treatment of skin cancers, melanomas, moles, and other tumors of the skin, the management of contact dermatitis, and other allergic and nonallergic skin disorders, and in the recognition of the skin manifestations of systemic (including internal malignancy) and infectious diseases. Dermatologists have special training in dermatopathology and in the surgical techniques used in dermatology. They also have expertise in the management of cosmetic disorders of the skin, such as hair loss and scars, and the skin changes associated with aging.

Training required: four years

Subspecialties
- *Clinical and laboratory dermatological immunology* This dermatologist utilizes various specialized laboratory procedures to diagnose disorders characterized by defective responses of the body's immune system. Immunodermatologists also may provide consultation in the management of these disorders and administer specialized forms of therapy for these diseases.

- *Dermatopathology* A dermatopathologist has the expertise to diagnose and monitor diseases of the skin, including infectious, immunologists, degenerative, and neoplastic disease. This entails the examination and interpretation of specially prepared tissue sections, cellular scrapings, and smears of skin lesions by means of routine and special (electron and fluorescent) microscopes.

EMERGENCY MEDICINE

An emergency physician focuses on the immediate decision making and action necessary to prevent death or any further disability, both in the pre-hospital setting by directing emergency medical technicians and in the emergency department. The emergency physician provides immediate recognition, evaluation, care, stabilization, and disposition of a generally diversified population of adult and pediatric patients in response to acute illness or injury.

Training required: three years

Subspecialties

- *Medical toxicology* An emergency physician in this field has special knowledge about the evaluation and management of patients with accidental or purposeful poisoning through exposure to prescription and nonprescription medications, drugs of abuse, household or industrial toxins, and environmental toxins. Areas of medical toxicology include acute pediatric and adult drug ingestion; drug abuse, addictions and withdrawal; chemical poisoning exposure and toxicity; hazardous materials exposure and toxicity; and occupational toxicology.

- *Pediatric emergency medicine* A pediatric emergency physician has special qualifications to manage emergencies in infants and children.

- *Sports medicine* An emergency physician in this field has special knowledge in sports medicine and is responsible for continuous care in the field of sports medicine, not only for the enhancement of health and fitness, but also for the prevention and management of injury and illness. A sports medicine physician has knowledge and experience in the promotion of wellness and the role of exercise in promoting a healthy lifestyle. Knowledge of exercise physiology, biomechanics, nutrition, psychology, physical rehabilitation, and epidemiology is essential to the practice of sports medicine.

- *Undersea and hyperbaric medicine* This emergency medicine physician, with additional and specialized training, has expertise in the treatment of decompression illness and diving accident cases and uses hyperbaric oxygen therapy treatment for conditions such as carbon monoxide poisoning, gas gangrene, nonhealing wounds, tissue damage from radiation and burns, and bone infections. This specialist also serves as consultant to other physicians in all aspects of hyperbaric chamber operations, and assesses risks and applies appropriate standards to prevent disease and disability in divers and other people working in altered atmospheric conditions.

FAMILY PRACTICE

A family physician is concerned with the total health care of the individual and the family, and is trained to diagnose and treat a wide variety of ailments in patients of all ages. The family physician receives a broad range of training that includes internal medicine, pediatrics, obstetrics and gynecology, psychiatry, and geriatrics. Special emphasis is placed on prevention and the primary care of entire families, utilizing consultations and community resources when appropriate.

Training required: three years

Subspecialties

Certification in one of the following subspecialties requires additional training and examination.

- *Geriatric medicine* This family practice physician has special knowledge of the aging process and special skills in the diagnostic, therapeutic, preventative, and rehabilitative aspects of illness in the elderly. This specialist cares for geriatric patients in the patient's home, the office, or long-term care settings such as nursing homes and the hospital.

- *Sports medicine* This family practice physician is trained to be responsible for continuous care in the field of sports medicine, not only for the enhancement of health and fitness, but also for the prevention of injury and illness. A sports medicine physician must have knowledge and experience in the promotion of wellness and the prevention of injury. Knowledge about special areas of medicine such as exercise physiology, biomechanics, nutrition psychology, physical rehabilitation, epidemiology, physical evaluation, injuries (treatment and prevention and referral practice), and the role of exercise in promoting a healthy lifestyle are essential to the practice of sports medicine. The sports medicine physician requires special education to provide the knowledge to improve the health care of the individual engaged in physical exercise (sports), whether as an individual or in team participation.

INTERNAL MEDICINE

An internist is a personal physician who provides long-term, comprehensive care in the office and the hospital, managing both common and complex illness of adolescents, adults, and the elderly. Internists are trained in the diagnosis and treatment of cancer, infections, and diseases affecting the heart, blood, kidneys, joints, and digestive, respiratory, and vascular systems. They are also trained in the essentials of primary care internal medicine, which incorporates an understanding of disease prevention, wellness, substance abuse, mental health, and effective treatment of common problems of the eyes, ears, skin, nervous system, and reproductive organs.

Training required: three years

Subspecialties
Certification in one of the following subspecialties requires additional training and examination.

- *Adolescent medicine* An internist who specializes in adolescent medicine is a multidisciplinary health care specialist trained in the unique physical, psychological, and social characteristics of adolescents, their health care problems, and their needs.

- *Cardiovascular disease* The internist specializes in diseases of the heart, lungs, and blood vessels and manages complex cardiac conditions such as heart attacks and life-threatening, abnormal heartbeat rhythms.

- *Interventional cardiology* An internist in this subspecialty of cardiology uses specialized imaging and other diagnostic techniques to evaluate blood flow and pressure in the coronary arteries and chambers of the heart, and technical procedures and medications to treat abnormalities that impair the function of the heart.

- *Clinical cardiac electrophysiology* This field of special interest within the subspecialty of cardiovascular disease involves intricate technical procedures to evaluate heart rhythms and determine appropriate treatment for them.

- *Clinical and laboratory immunology* This internist uses laboratory tests and complex procedures to diagnose and treat disorders characterized by defective responses to the body's immune system.

- *Critical care medicine* The internist diagnoses, treats, and supports patients with multiple organ dysfunction. This specialist may have administrative responsibilities for intensive care units, and may also facilitate and coordinate patient care among the primary physician, the critical care staff, and other specialties.

- *Endocrinology, diabetes, and metabolism* This internist concentrates on disorders of the internal (endocrine) glands such as the thyroid and adrenal glands. The specialist also deals with diabetes, metabolic and nutritional disorders, pituitary diseases, and menstrual and sexual problems.

- *Gastroenterology* An internist in this field specializes in diagnosis and treatment of diseases of the digestive organs including the stomach, bowels, liver, and gallbladder. This specialist treats conditions such as abdominal pain, ulcers, diarrhea, cancer, and jaundice, and performs complex diagnostic and therapeutic procedures using endoscopes to see internal organs.

- *Geriatric medicine* An internist with special knowledge of the aging process uses special skills in the diagnostic, therapeutic, preventive, and rehabilitative aspects of illness in the elderly. This specialist cares for geriatric patients in the patient's home, the office, long-term care settings such as nursing homes, and the hospital.

- *Hematology* An internist with this subspecialty specializes in diseases of the blood, spleen, and lymph glands. This specialist treats conditions such as anemia, clotting disorders, sickle cell disease, hemophilia, leukemia, and lymphoma.

- *Infectious disease* This internist deals with infectious diseases of all types and in all organs. Conditions requiring selective use of antibiotics call for this special skill. This physician often diagnoses and treats AIDS patients and patients with fevers that have not been explained. Infectious disease specialists may also have expertise in preventive medicine and conditions associated with travel.

- *Medical oncology* A medical oncologist is an internist who specializes in the diagnosis and treatment of all types of cancer and other benign and malignant tumors. This specialist decides on and administers chemotherapy for malignancy, as well as consulting with surgeons and radiotherapists on other treatments for cancer.

- *Nephrology* An internist in this field treats high blood pressure and disorders of the kidney, maintains fluid and mineral balance, and performs dialysis of body wastes when the kidneys do not function. This specialist consults with surgeons about kidney transplantation.

- *Pulmonary disease* An internist in this field treats disease of the lungs and airways. This pulmonologist diagnoses and treats cancer, pneumonia, pleurisy, asthma, occupational diseases, bronchitis, sleep disorders, emphysema, and other complex disorders of the lungs.

- *Rheumatology* A rheumatologist is an internist who treats disease of joints, muscle, bones, and tendons. This specialist diagnoses and treats arthritis, back pain, muscle strains, common athletic injuries, and collagen diseases.

- *Sports medicine* This is a family practice physician who is trained to be responsible for continuous care in the field of sports medicine, not only for the enhancement of health and fitness, but also for the prevention of injury and illness. A sports medicine physician must have knowledge and experience in the promotion of wellness and the prevention of injury. Knowledge about special areas of medicine such as exercise physiology, biomechanics, nutrition psychology, physical rehabilitation, epidemiology, physical evaluation, injuries (treatment and prevention, and referral practice), and the role of exercise in promoting a healthy lifestyle are essential to the practice of sports medicine. The sports medicine physician requires special education to provide the knowledge to improve the health care of the individual engaged in physical exercise (sports) whether as an individual or in team participation.

MEDICAL GENETICS

A specialist in medical genetics is trained in diagnostic and therapeutic procedures for patients with genetically linked diseases. This specialist uses modern cytogenetic, radiologic, and biochemical testing to assist in specialized genetic counseling; implements needed therapeutic interventions; and provides prevention through prenatal diagnosis.

A medical geneticist plans and coordinates large-scale screening programs for inborn errors of metabolism, hemoglobinopathies, chromosome abnormalities, and neural tube defects.

Training required: two years

Certificates

The Board issues multiple general certificates in the following areas of genetics.

- *Clinical biochemical genetics* A clinical biochemical geneticist demonstrates competence in performing and interpreting biochemical analyses relevant to the diagnosis and management of human genetic diseases, and is a consultant regarding laboratory diagnosis of a broad range of inherited disorders.

- *Clinical cytogenetics* A clinical cytogeneticist demonstrates competence in providing laboratory diagnostic and clinical interpretive services dealing with cellular components, particularly chromosomes, associated with heredity.

- *Clinical genetics (M.D.)* A clinical geneticist demonstrates competence in providing comprehensive diagnostic, management, and counseling services for genetic disorders.

- *Clinical molecular genetics* A clinical molecular geneticist demonstrates competence in performing and interpreting molecular analyses relevant to the diagnosis and management of human genetic diseases, and is consultant regarding laboratory diagnosis of a broad range of inherited disorders.

- *Ph.D. medical genetics* A medical geneticist works in association with medical specialists, is affiliated with a clinical genetics program, and serves as a consultant to medical and dental specialists.

Subspecialty

Certification in molecular genetic pathology requires one year additional training and examination.

- *Molecular genetic pathology* A molecular genetic pathologist is expert in the principles, theories, and technologies of molecular biology and molecular genetics. This expertise is used to make or confirm diagnoses of Mendelian genetic disorders, of human development, and infectious diseases and malignancies, and to assess the natural history of those disorders. A molecular genetic pathologist provides information about gene structure, function, and alteration, and applies laboratory techniques for diagnosis, treatment, and prognosis for individuals with related disorders.

NEUROLOGICAL SURGERY

A neurological surgeon provides the operative and nonoperative management (i.e., prevention, diagnosis, evaluation, treatment, critical care, and rehabilitation) of disorders of the central, peripheral, and autonomic nervous systems, including their supporting structures and vascular supply; the evaluation and treatment of pathological processes that modify function or activity of the nervous system; and the operative and nonoperative management of pain. A neurological surgeon treats patients with disorders of the nervous system; disorders of the brain, meninges, skull, and their blood supply, including the extracranial carotid and vertebral arteries; disorders of the pituitary gland; disorders of the spinal cord, meninges, and vertebral column, including those that may require treatment by spinal fusion or instrumentation; and disorders of the cranial and spinal nerves throughout their distribution.

Training required: seven years (including general surgery)

Neurology/Child Neurology

A neurologist specializes in the diagnosis and treatment of all types of disease or impaired function of the brain, spinal cord, peripheral nerves, muscles, and autonomic nervous system, as well as the blood vessels that relate to these structures. A child neurologist has special skills in the diagnosis and management of neurologic disorders of the neonatal period, infancy, early childhood, and adolescence.

Subspecialties Requiring Additional Training

Certification in one of the following subspecialties requires an additional four years of training and examination.

- *Clinical neurophysiology* A neurologist who specializes in the diagnosis and management of central, peripheral, and autonomic nervous system disorders using a combination of clinical evaluation and electrophysiologic testing such as electroencephalography (EEG), electromyography (EMG), and the nerve conduction studies (NCS), among others.

- *Neurodevelopmental disabilities* A pediatrician or neurologist in this field specializes in the diagnosis and management of chronic conditions that affect the developing and mature nervous system such as cerebral palsy, mental retardation, chronic behavioral syndromes, and neurologic conditions.

- *Pain medicine* A neurologist in this field provides a high level of care, either as a primary physician or consultant, for patients experiencing problems with acute, chronic, or cancer pain in both hospital and ambulatory settings. Patient care needs may also be coordinated with other specialties.

NUCLEAR MEDICINE

A nuclear medicine specialist employs the properties of radioactive atoms and molecules in the diagnosis and treatment of disease, and in research. Radiation detection and imaging instrument systems are used to detect disease as it changes the function and metabolism of normal cells, tissues, and organs. A wide variety of diseases can be found in this way, usually before the structure of the organ involved by the disease can be seen to be abnormal by any other techniques. Early detection of coronary artery disease (including acute heart attack), early cancer detection and evaluation of the effect of tumor treatment, diagnosis of infection and inflammation anywhere in the body, and early detection of blood clot in the lungs are all possible with these techniques. Unique forms of radioactive molecules can attack and kill cancer cells (e.g., lymphoma and thyroid cancer) or can relieve the severe pain of cancer that has spread to bone.

The nuclear medicine specialist has special knowledge in the biologic effects of radiation exposure, the fundamentals of the physical sciences, and the principles and operation of radiation detection and imaging instrumentation systems.

Training required: three years

OBSTETRICS AND GYNECOLOGY

An obstetrician/gynecologist possesses special knowledge, skills, and professional capability in the medical and surgical care of the female reproductive system and associated disorders. This physician serves as a consultant to other physicians and as a primary physician for women.

Training required: four years, plus two years in clinical practice before certification is complete

Subspecialties
Certification in one of the following subspecialties requires additional training and examination.

- *Critical care medicine* An obstetrician-gynecologist who specializes in critical care medicine diagnoses, treats, and supports female patients with multiple organ dysfunction. This specialist may have administrative responsibilities for intensive care units, and may also facilitate and coordinate patient care among the primary physician, the critical care staff, and other specialists.

- *Gynecologic oncology* An obstetrician-gynecologist with this sub-specialty provides consultation and comprehensive management of patients with gynecologic cancer, including those diagnostic and therapeutic procedures necessary for total care of the patient with gynecologic cancer and resulting complications.

- *Maternal-fetal medicine* An obstetrician-gynecologist who cares for or provides consultation to patients with complications during pregnancy. This specialist has advanced knowledge of the obstetrical, medical, and surgical complications of pregnancy, and their effect on both the mother and the fetus. He or she also possesses expertise in the most current diagnostic and treatment modalities used in the care of patients with complicated pregnancies.

- *Reproductive endocrinology* An obstetrician-gynecologist in this field is capable of managing complex problems relating to reproductive endocrinology and infertility.

OPHTHALMOLOGY

An ophthalmologist has the knowledge and professional skills needed to provide comprehensive eye and vision care. Ophthalmologists are medically trained to diagnose, monitor, and medically or surgically treat all ocular and visual disorders. This includes problems affecting the eye and its component structures, the eyelids, the orbit, and the visual pathways. In so doing, an ophthalmologist prescribes vision services, including glasses and contact lenses.

Training required: four years

ORTHOPEDIC SURGERY

An orthopedic surgeon is trained in the preservation, investigation, and restoration of the form and function of the extremities, of the spine and associated structures by medical, surgical, and physical means.

An orthopedic surgeon is involved with the care of children or adult patients whose musculoskeletal system has deformities or injuries, or who have a degenerative disease of the spine, hands, feet, knee, hip, shoulder, and elbow. An orthopedic surgeon is also concerned with primary and secondary muscular problems and the effects of central or peripheral nervous system lesions of the musculoskeletal system.

Training required: five years (including general surgery training) plus two years in clinical practice before final certification is achieved

OTOLARYNGOLOGY

An otolaryngologist—head and neck surgeon—provides comprehensive medical and surgical care for patients with diseases and disorders that affect the ears, nose, throat, the respiratory and upper alimentary systems, and related structures of the head and neck.

An otolaryngologist diagnoses and provides medical and/or surgical therapy or prevention of diseases; allergies; neoplasms; deformities; disorders and/or injuries of the ears, nose, sinuses, throat, respiratory and upper alimentary systems, face, jaws, and the other head and neck systems. Head and neck oncology, facial plastic and reconstructive surgery, and the treatment of disorders on hearing and voices are fundamental areas of expertise.

Training required: five years

Subspecialties
Certification in one of the following subspecialties requires additional training and examination.

- *Otology/neurology* This type of otolaryngologist treats disease of the ear and temporal bone, including disorders of hearing and balance. The additional training in otology and neurology emphasizes the study of embryology, anatomy, physiology, epidemiology, pathophysiology, pathology, genetics, immunology, microbiology, and the etiology of diseases of the ear and temporal bone.

- *Pediatric otolaryngology* A pediatric otolaryngologist has special expertise in the management of infants and children with disorders that include congenital and acquired conditions involving the aerodigestive tract, nose and paranasal sinuses, the ear, and other

areas of the head and neck. The pediatric otolaryngologist has special skills in the diagnosis, treatment, and management of childhood
disorders of voice, speech, language, and hearing.

- *Plastic surgery within the head and neck* An otolaryngologist with
  additional training in plastic and reconstructive procedures specializes in treatment of the head, face, neck, and associated structures,
  including cutaneous head and neck oncology and reconstruction,
  management of maxillofacial trauma, soft tissue repair, and neural
  surgery. The field is diverse and involves a wide age range of patients,
  from the newborn to the aged. Although both cosmetic and reconstructive surgery are practiced, there are many additional procedures
  that interface with them.

PATHOLOGY

A pathologist deals with the causes and nature of disease and contributes
to diagnosis, prognosis, and treatment through knowledge gained by the
laboratory application of the biologic, chemical, and physical sciences.

A pathologist uses information gathered from the microscopic examination of tissue specimens, cells, and body fluids, and from clinical laboratory tests on body fluids and secretions for the diagnosis, exclusion, and
monitoring of disease.

Training required: five to seven years

Subspecialties
Certification in one of the following subspecialties requires additional
training and examination.

- *Blood banking/transfusion medicine* A physician who specializes in
  blood banking/transfusion medicine is responsible for the maintenance of an adequate blood supply, blood donor and patient-recipient
  safety, and appropriate blood utilization. Pretransfusion compatibil-
  ity testing and antibody testing assure that blood transfusions, when
  indicated, are as safe as possible. This physician directs the prepara-
  tion and safe use of specially prepared blood components, including
  red blood cells, white blood cells, platelets, and plasma constituents.

- *Chemical pathology* A chemical pathologist has expertise in the biochemistry of the human body as it applies to the understanding of the cause and progress of disease. This physician functions as a clinical consultant in the diagnosis and treatment of human disease. Chemical pathology entails the application of biochemical data to the detection, confirmation, or monitoring of disease.

- *Cytopathology* A cytopathologist is an anatomic pathologist trained in the diagnosis of human disease by means of the study of cells obtained from body secretions and fluids, by scraping, washing, or sponging the surface of a lesion, or by the aspiration of a tumor mass or body organ with a fine needle. A major aspect of a cytopathologist's practice is the interpretation of Papanicolaou-stained smears of cells from the female reproductive systems, the Pap test. However, the cytopathologist's expertise is applied to the diagnosis of cells from all systems and areas of the body. He or she is a consultant to all medical specialists.

- *Dermatopathology* A dermatopathologist is expert in diagnosing and monitoring diseases of the skin, including infectious, immunologic, degenerative, and neoplastic diseases. This entails the examination and interpretation of specially prepared tissue sections, cellular scrapings, and smears of skin lesions by means of light microscopy, electron microscopy, and fluorescence microscopy.

- *Forensic pathology* A forensic pathologist is expert in investigating and evaluating cases of sudden, unexpected, suspicious, and violent death, as well as other specific classes of death defined by law. The forensic pathologist serves the public as coroner or medical examiner, or by performing medicolegal autopsies for such officials.

- *Hematology* A hematologist physician who is expert in diseases that affect blood cells, blood clotting mechanisms, bone marrow, and lymph nodes. He or she has the knowledge and technical skills essential for the laboratory diagnosis of anemias, leukemias, lymphomas, bleeding disorders, and blood clotting disorders.

- *Medical microbiology* A physician who is expert in the isolation and identification of microbial agents that cause infectious disease. Viruses, bacteria, and fungi, as well as parasites, are identified and, where possible, tested for susceptibility to appropriate antimicrobial agents.

- *Molecular genetic pathology* A molecular genetic pathologist is expert in the principles, theory, and technologies of molecular biology and molecular genetics. This expertise is used to make or confirm diagnoses of Mendelian genetic disorders, disorders of human development, infectious diseases and malignancies, and to assess the natural history of those disorders. A molecular genetic pathologist provides information about gene structure, functions, and alteration, and applies laboratory techniques for diagnosis, treatment, and prognosis for individuals with related disorders.

- *Neuropathology* A neuropathologist is expert in the diagnosis of diseases of the nervous system and skeletal muscles and functions as a consultant primarily to neurologists and neurosurgeons. The neuropathologist is knowledgeable in the infirmities of humans as they affect the nervous and neuromuscular systems, be they degenerative infectious, metabolic, immunologic, neoplastic, vascular, or physical in nature.

- *Pediatric pathology* A pediatric pathologist is expert in the laboratory diagnosis of diseases that occur during fetal growth, infancy, and child development. The practice requires a strong foundation in general pathology and substantial understanding of normal growth and development, along with extensive knowledge of pediatric medicine.

PEDIATRICS

A pediatrician is concerned with the physical, emotional, and social health of children from birth to young adulthood. Care encompasses a broad spectrum of health services ranging from preventive health care to the diagnosis and treatment of acute and chronic diseases.

A pediatrician deals with biological, social, and environmental influences on the developing child, and with the impact of disease and dysfunction on development.

Training required: three years

Subspecialties

Certification in one of the following subspecialties requires additional training and examination.

- *Adolescent medicine* A pediatrician who specializes in adolescent medicine is a multidisciplinary health care specialist trained in the unique physical, psychological, and social characteristics of adolescents, their health care problems, and their needs.

- *Clinical and laboratory immunology* A pediatrician in this field utilizes laboratory tests and complex procedures to diagnose and treat disorders characterized by defective responses of the body's immune system.

- *Developmental-behavioral pediatrics* A developmental-behavioral specialist is a pediatrician with special training and experience who aims to foster understanding and promotion of optimal development of children and advocacy efforts. This physician assists in the prevention, diagnosis, and management of developmental difficulties and problematic behaviors in children, and in the family dysfunctions that compromise children's development.

- *Medical toxicology* A pediatrician with this specialty focuses on the evaluation and management of patients with accidental or intentional poisoning through exposure to prescriptions and nonprescription medications, drugs of abuse, household or industrial toxins, and environmental toxins. Important areas of medical toxicology include acute pediatric and adult drug ingestion; drug abuse, addiction, and withdrawal; chemical poisoning exposure and toxicity; hazardous materials exposure and toxicity; and occupational toxicology.

- *Neonatal-perinatal medicine* A pediatrician in this field is the principal care provider for sick newborn infants. Clinical expertise is used for direct patient care and for consulting with obstetrical colleagues to plan for the care of mothers who have high-risk pregnancies.

- *Neurodevelopmental disabilities* This pediatrician treats children having developmental delays or learning disorders, including those associated with visual and hearing impairment, mental retardation, cerebral palsy, spina bifida, autism, and other chronic neurologic conditions. This specialist provides medical consultation and education and assumes leadership in the interdisciplinary management of children with neurodevelopmental disorders. They may also focus on the early identification and diagnosis of neurodevelopmental disabilities in infants and young children, as well as on changes that occur as the child with developmental disabilities grows.

- *Pediatric cardiology* A pediatrician cardiologist provides comprehensive care to patients with cardiovascular problems. This specialist is skilled in selecting, performing, and evaluating the structural and functional assessment of the heart and blood vessels, and the clinical evaluation of cardiovascular disease.

- *Pediatric critical care medicine* This pediatrician is expert in advanced life support for children from term or near-term neonate to the adolescent. This competence extends to the critical care management of life-threatening organ systems failure from any cause in both medical and surgical patients, and to the support of vital physiological functions. This specialist may have administrative responsibilities for intensive care units and also facilitate patient care among other specialists.

- *Pediatric emergency medicine* This pediatrician has special qualifications to manage emergencies in infants and children.

- *Pediatric endocrinology* This pediatrician provides expert care to infants, children, and adolescents who have diseases that result from an abnormality in the endocrine glands (glands that secrete hormones). These diseases include diabetes mellitus, growth failure, unusual size for age, early or late pubertal development, birth defects, the genital region, and disorders of the thyroid, and the adrenal and pituitary glands.

- *Pediatric gastroenterology* A pediatrician in this field specializes in the diagnosis and treatment of diseases of the digestive systems of infants, children, and adolescents. This specialist treats conditions such as abdominal pain, ulcers, diarrhea, cancer, and jaundice, and performs complex diagnostic and therapeutic procedures using lighted scopes to see internal organs.

- *Pediatric hematology-oncology* A pediatrician trained in the combination of pediatrics, hematology, and oncology uses this skill to recognize and manage pediatric blood disorders and cancerous diseases.

- *Pediatric infectious diseases* A pediatrician trained in this field cares for children in the diagnosis, treatment, and prevention of infectious diseases. This specialist can apply specific knowledge to affect a better outcome for pediatric infections with complicated courses, underlying diseases that predispose to unusual or severe infections, unclear diagnoses, uncommon diseases, and complex or investigational treatments.

- *Pediatric nephrology* A pediatrician in this field deals with the normal and abnormal development and maturation of the kidney and urinary tract, the mechanisms by which the kidney can be damaged, the evaluation and treatment of renal disease, fluid and electrolyte abnormalities, hypertension, and renal replacement therapy.

- *Pediatric pulmonology* A pediatric pulmonologist is dedicated to the prevention and treatment of all respiratory diseases affecting infants, children, and young adults. This specialist is knowledgeable about the growth and development of the lung, and assessment of respiratory function in infants and children. He or she is experienced in a variety of invasive and noninvasive diagnostic techniques.

- *Pediatric rheumatology* A pediatrician in this field treats diseases of joints, muscle, bones, and tendons. A pediatric rheumatologist diagnoses and treats arthritis, back pain, muscle strains, common athlete injuries, and "collagen" diseases.

- *Sports medicine* This pediatrician is responsible for continuous care in the field of sports medicine, not only for the enhancement of health and fitness, but also for the prevention of injury and illness. A sports medicine physician must have knowledge and experience in the promotion of wellness and the prevention of injury. Knowledge about special areas of medicine such as exercise physiology, biomechanics, nutrition, psychology, physical rehabilitation, epidemiology, physical evaluation, injuries (treatment and prevention and referral practice), and the role of exercise in promoting a healthy lifestyle is essential

to the practice of sports medicine. The sports medicine physician requires special education to provide the knowledge to improve the health care of the individual engaged in physical exercise (sports), whether as an individual or in team participation.

PHYSICAL MEDICINE AND REHABILITATION

Physical medicine and rehabilitation, also referred to as rehabilitation medicine, is the medical specialty concerned with diagnosing, evaluating, and treating patients with physical disabilities. These disabilities may arise from conditions affecting the musculoskeletal systems such as neck and back pain, sports injuries, or other painful conditions affecting the limbs—for example, carpal tunnel syndrome. Alternatively, the disabilities may result from neurological trauma or disease such as spinal cord injury or stroke.

A physician certified in physical medicine and rehabilitation is often called a physiatrist. The primary goal of the physiatrist is to achieve maximal restoration of physical, psychological, social, and vocational function through comprehensive rehabilitation. Pain management is often an important part of the role of the physiatrist. For diagnosis and evaluation, a physiatrist may include the techniques of electromyography to supplement the standard history, physical, X-ray, and laboratory examinations. The physiatrist has expertise in the appropriate use of therapeutic exercise, prosthetics (artificial limbs), orthotics, and mechanical and electrical devices.

Training required: four years plus one year of clinical practice

Subspecialties
Certification in one of the following subspecialties requires additional training and examination.

- *Pain medicine* A physician with this certification provides a high level of care, either as a primary physician or consultant, for patients experiencing problems with acute, chronic, or cancer pain in both hospital and ambulatory settings.

- *Pediatric rehabilitation medicine* This physiatrist utilizes an interdisciplinary approach and addresses the prevention, diagnosis, treatment, and management of congenital and childhood onset physical impairments including related or secondary medical, physical, functional, psychosocial, and vocational limitations or conditions, with an understanding of the life course of disability. This physician is trained in the identification of functional capabilities and selections of the best rehabilitation intervention strategies with an understanding of the continuum of care.

- *Spinal cord injury medicine* A physician who addresses the prevention, diagnosis, treatment, and management of traumatic spinal cord injury and nontraumatic etiologies of spinal cord dysfunction by working in an interdisciplinary manner. Care is provided to patients of all ages on a lifelong basis and covers related medical, physical, psychological, and vocational disabilities and complications.

PLASTIC SURGERY

A plastic surgeon deals with the repair, reconstruction, or replacement of physical defects of form or function involving the skin, musculoskeletal system, craniomaxillofacial structures, hand, extremities, breast and trunk, and external genitalia. The surgeon uses aesthetic surgical principles not only to improve undesirable qualities of normal structures but in all reconstructive procedures as well.

A plastic surgeon possesses special knowledge and skill in the design and surgery of grafts, flaps, free tissue transfer, and replantation. Competence in the management of complex wounds, the use of implantable materials, and tumor surgery is required.

Training required: five to seven years

Specialties
Certification in one of the following subspecialties requires additional training and examination.

- *Plastic surgery within the head and neck* A plastic surgeon in this field has additional training in plastic and reconstructive procedures within the head, face, neck, and associated structures, including cutaneous head and neck oncology and reconstruction, management of maxillofacial trauma, soft tissue repair and neural surgery. The field is diverse and involves a wide age range of patients, from the newborn to the aged. Both cosmetic and reconstructive surgery are practiced, but there are many additional procedures that interfere with them.
- *Surgery of the hand* This plastic surgeon has additional training in the investigation, preservation, and restoration by medical, surgical, and rehabilitative means of all structures of the upper extremity directly affecting the form and function of the hand and wrist.

PREVENTIVE MEDICINE

A preventive medicine specialist focuses on the health of individuals and defined populations in order to protect, promote, and maintain health and well-being, and to prevent disease, disability, and premature death. There are seven distinctive components of preventive medicine:

1. Biostatistics and the application of biostatistical principles and methodology
2. Epidemiology and its application to population-based medicine and research
3. Health services management and administration, including developing, assessing, and assuring health policies; planning, implementing, directing, budgeting, and evaluating population health and disease management programs; and utilizing legislative and regulatory processes to enhance health
4. Control of environmental factors that may adversely affect health
5. Control and prevention of occupational factors that may adversely affect health safety

6. Clinical preventive medicine activities, including measures to promote health and prevent the occurrence, progression, and disabling effects of disease and injury

7. Assessment of social, cultural, and behavioral influences on health

A preventive medicine physician may be a specialist in general preventive medicine, public health, occupational medicine, or aerospace medicine. This specialist works with large population groups as well as with individual patients to promote health and help them understand the risks of disease, injury, disability, and death, seeking to modify and eliminate these risks.

Training required: three years

Subspecialties
Certification in one of the following subspecialties requires additional training and examination.

- *Medical toxicology* This specialist is expert in the evaluation and management of patients with accidental or intentional poisoning through exposure to prescription and nonprescription medications, drugs of abuse, household or industrial toxins, and environmental toxins. Important areas of medical toxicology include acute pediatric and adult drug ingestion; drug abuse, addictions, and withdrawal; chemical poisoning exposure and toxicity; hazardous materials exposure and toxicity; and occupational toxicology.

- *Undersea and hyperbaric medicine* A specialist in this field treats decompression illness and diving accident cases and uses hyperbaric oxygen therapy to treat such conditions as carbon monoxide poisoning, gas gangrene, nonhealing wounds, tissue damage from radiation and burns, and bone infections. This specialist also serves as consultant to other physicians in all aspects of hyperbaric chamber operations, and assesses risks and applies appropriate standards to prevent disease and disability in divers and other persons working in altered atmospheric conditions.

PSYCHIATRY

A psychiatrist specializes in the prevention, diagnosis, and treatment of mental, addictive, and emotional disorders such as schizophrenia and other psychotic disorders, mood disorders, anxiety disorders, substance-related disorders, sexual and gender identity disorders, and adjustment disorders. The psychiatrist is able to understand the biologic, psychologic, and social components of illness, and therefore is uniquely prepared to treat the whole person. A psychiatrist is qualified to order diagnostic laboratory tests and to prescribe medications, evaluate and treat psychologic and interpersonal problems, and to intervene with families who are coping with stress, crisis, and other problems in living.

Training required: four years

Subspecialties
Certification in one of the following subspecialties requires additional training and examination.

- *Addiction psychiatry* An addiction psychiatrist who focuses on the evaluation and treatment of individuals with alcohol, drug, or other substance-related disorders and of individuals with dual diagnosis of substance-related and other psychiatric disorders.

- *Child and adolescent psychiatry* A child and adolescent psychiatrist with additional training in the diagnosis and treatment of developmental, behavioral, emotional, and mental disorders of childhood and adolescence.

- *Clinical neurophysiology* This type of psychiatrist has expertise in the diagnosis and management of central, peripheral, and autonomic nervous system disorders and uses a combination of clinical evaluation and electrophysiologic testing, such as electroencephalography (EEG), electromyography (EMG), and nerve conduction studies (NCS).

- *Forensic psychiatry* A psychiatrist in this field focuses on the interrelationships between psychiatry and civil, criminal, and administrative law. This specialist evaluates individuals involved with the legal system and provides specialized treatment to those incarcerated in jails, prisons, and forensic psychiatry hospitals.

- *Geriatric psychiatry* A psychiatrist in this field has expertise in the prevention, evaluation, diagnosis, and treatment of mental and emotional disorders in the elderly. The geriatric psychiatrist seeks to improve the psychiatric care of the elderly both in health and in disease.

- *Pain medicine* A psychiatrist with this specialty provides a high level of care, either as a primary physician or consultant, for patients experiencing problems with acute, chronic, or cancer pain in both hospital and ambulatory settings. Patient care needs may also be coordinated with other specialists.

RADIOLOGY

A radiologist utilizes radiologic methodologies to diagnose and treat disease. Physicians practicing in the field of radiology most often specialize in radiology, diagnostic radiology, radiation oncology, or radiological physics.

- *Diagnostic radiology* This type of radiologist utilizes X-ray, radionuclides, ultrasound, and electromagnetic radiation to diagnose and treat disease.

- *Radiation oncology* A radiologist in this field deals with the therapeutic applications of radiant energy and its modifiers and the study and management of disease, especially malignant tumors.

- *Radiological physics* A radiological physicist deals with the diagnostic and therapeutic applications of roentgen rays, gamma rays from sealed sources, ultrasonic radiation, and radio-frequency radiation, as well as the equipment associated with their production and use, including radiation safety.

Training required: four years

Subspecialties
Certification in one of the following subspecialties requires additional training and examination.

- *Neuroradiology* A radiologist in this field diagnoses and treats diseases utilizing imaging procedures as they relate to the brain, spine and spinal cord, head, neck, and organs of special sense in adults and children.

- *Nuclear radiology* A nuclear radiologist is involved in the analysis and imaging of radionuclides and radio-labeled substances in vitro and in vivo for diagnosis, and the administration of radionuclides and radio-labeled substances for the treatment of disease.

- *Pediatric radiology* A pediatric radiologist is proficient in all forms of diagnostic imaging as it pertains to the treatment of diseases in the newborn, infant, child, and adolescent. This specialist has knowledge of both imaging and interventional procedures related to the care and management of diseases of children. A pediatric radiologist must be highly knowledgeable of all organ systems as they relate to growth and development, congenital malformations, diseases peculiar to infants and children, and diseases that begin in childhood but cause substantial residual impairment in adulthood.

- *Vascular and interventional radiology* A radiologist with this specialty diagnoses and treats diseases by various radiologic imaging modalities. These include fluoroscopy, digital radiography, computed tomography, sonography, and magnetic resonance imaging.

GENERAL SURGERY

A general surgeon manages a broad spectrum of surgical conditions affecting almost any area of the body. The surgeon establishes the diagnosis and provides the preoperative, operative, and postoperative care to surgical patients and is usually responsible for the comprehensive management of the trauma victim and the critically ill surgical patient.

The surgeon uses a variety of diagnostic techniques, including endoscopy, for observing internal structures, and may use specialized instruments during operative procedures. A general surgeon is expected to be familiar with the salient features of other surgical specialties in order to recognize problems in those areas and to know when to refer a patient to another specialist.

Training required: five years

Subspecialties
Certification in one of the following subspecialties requires additional training and examination.

- *Pediatric surgery* A surgeon with this specialty has expertise in the management of surgical conditions in premature and newborn infants, children, and adolescents.
- *Surgery of the hand* This surgeon has expertise in the investigation, preservation, and restoration by medical, surgical, and rehabilitative means, of all structures of the upper extremity directly affecting the form and functions of the hand and wrist.
- *Surgical critical care* This surgeon has expertise in the management of the critically ill and postoperative patient, particularly the trauma victim, and specializes in critical care medicine diagnoses, and treats and supports patients with multiple organ dysfunction. This specialist may have administrative responsibilities for intensive care units and may also facilitate and coordinate patient care among the primary physician, the critical care staff, and other specialists.
- *Vascular surgery* This surgeon has expertise in the management of surgical disorders of the blood vessels, excluding the intercranial vessels or the heart.

THORACIC SURGERY

A thoracic surgeon provides the operative, perioperative, and critical care of patients with pathologic conditions within the chest. Included is the surgical care of coronary artery disease; cancers of the lung, esophagus, and chest wall; abnormalities of the trachea; abnormalities of the great vessels and heart valves; congenital anomalies; tumors of the mediastinum; and diseases of the diaphragm. The management of the airway and injuries of the chest is within the scope of this specialty.

Thoracic surgeons have the knowledge, experience, and technical skills to accurately diagnose, operate upon sagely, and effectively manage patients with thoracic diseases of the chest. This requires substantial knowledge of cardiorespiratory physiology and oncology, as well as capability in the use of heart assist devices, management of abnormal heart rhythms and drainage of the chest cavity, respiratory support systems, endoscopy, and invasive and noninvasive diagnostic techniques.

Training required: seven to eight years

UROLOGY

A urologist manages benign and malignant medical and surgical disorders of the genitourinary system and the adrenal gland. This specialist has comprehensive knowledge of and skills in endoscopic, percutaneous, and open surgery of congenital and acquired conditions of the urinary and reproductive systems and their continuous structures.

Training required: five years

Better Business Bureau

General complaints are appropriate to send to the Better Business Bureau. Go to the national site at www.bbb.org and click on your state to find a local chapter.

Joint Commission on Accreditation of Health Care Organizations (JCAHO)

JCAHO is an independent, not-for-profit organization with governance by a board of physicians, nurses, and consumers. JCAHO sets the standards by which health care quality is measured in the United States and around the world. Use this website, www.jcaho.org, to check facility accreditation and quality.

National Association of Insurance Commissioners

Visit www.naic.org for a state listing for the department of insurance. On this site you may lodge complaints or research insurance companies in business in your state.

The National Committee for Quality Assurance

Visit www.ncqa.org for report cards on the nation's managed care plans (or managed care insurance companies providing HMO and PPO coverage).

Office of Inspector General: Exclusions Database

Use www.oig.hhs.gov to research providers excluded from the government payor programs. You will also find a wealth of information pertaining to government programs such as Medicare and Medicaid.

Patient Advocate Foundation

The mission of the Patient Advocate Foundation is to seek to safeguard patients through effective mediation, assuring access to care, maintenance of employment, and financial stability. The foundation is a national nonprofit resource for patients and their family members. Visit www.patientadvocate.org or call 1-800-532-5274.

State Board of Medical Examiners

State listings are provided by the Federation of State Medical Boards at www.fsmb.org.

Your state board of medical examiners is the body to submit complaints pertaining to physicians.

EXHIBIT 7-2 STATE BOARD OF MEDICAL EXAMINERS

Alabama State Board of Medical Examiners Larry D. Dixon, Executive Administrator P.O. Box 946 Montgomery, AL 36101-0946 (street address: 848 Washington Ave., 36104) (334) 242-4116, (800) 227-2606 Fax: (334) 242-4155 www.albme.org	Alaska State Medical Board Leslie A. Gallant, Executive Administrator 550 West Seventh Ave., Ste. 1500 Anchorage, AK 99501 (907) 269-8163 Fax: (907) 269-8196 www.dced.state.ak.us/occ/pmed.htm	Arizona Medical Board Timothy C. Miller, Executive Director 9545 E. Doubletree Ranch Rd. Scottsdale, AZ 85258-5514 (480) 551-2700 Fax: (480) 551-2704 www.azmdboard.org
Arizona Board of Osteopathic Examiners in Medicine and Surgery Jack Confer, Executive Director 9535 East Doubletree Ranch Rd. Scottsdale, AZ 85258-5539 (480) 657-7703 Fax: (480) 657-7715 www.azosteoboard.org	Arkansas State Medical Board Peggy P. Cryer, Executive Secretary 2100 Riverfront Dr. Little Rock, AR 72202-1793 (501) 296-1802 Fax: (501) 603-3555 www.armedicalboard.org	Medical Board of California David T. Thornton, Executive Director 1426 Howe Ave., Ste. 54 Sacramento, CA 95825-3236 (916) 263-2382 Fax: (916) 263-2944 www.caldocinfo.ca.gov
Osteopathic Medical Board of California Linda J. Bergmann, Executive Director 2720 Gateway Oaks Dr., Ste. 350 Sacramento, CA 95833-3500 (916) 263-3100 Fax: (916) 263-3117 www.ombc.ca.gov	Colorado Board of Medical Examiners Susan Miller, Program Administrator 1560 Broadway, Ste. 1350 Denver, CO 80202-5140 (303) 894-7690 Fax: (303) 894-7692 www.dora.state.co.us/medical	Connecticut Medical Examining Board Jeff Kardys, Board Liaison P.O. Box 340308 Hartford, CT 06134-0308 (street address: 410 Capitol Ave., MS13PHO) (860) 509-6000 Fax: (860) 509-7553 Licensing Information: (860) 509-7563 www.dph.state.ct.us
Delaware Board of Medical Practice Gayle MacAfee, Executive Director P.O. Box 1401 Dover, DE 19903 (street address: 861 Silver Lake Blvd., Cannon Building, Ste. 203, 19904) (302) 739-4522 Fax: (302) 739-2711 www.professionallicensing.state.de.us	District of Columbia Board of Medicine James R. Granger, Jr., Executive Director 717 14th Street, NW Ste. 600 Washington DC 20005 (202) 724-4900 Fax: (202) 727-8471 www.dchealth.dc.gov	Florida Board of Medicine Larry McPherson, Executive Director Department of Health 4052 Bald Cypress Way, BIN #C03 Tallahassee, FL 32399-3253 (850) 245-4131 Fax: (850) 488-9325 www.doh.state.fl.us

Florida Board of Osteopathic Medicine
Pamela King, Executive Director
4052 Bald Cypress Way, BIN C06
Tallahassee, FL 32399-1753
(850) 245-4161
Fax: (850) 487-9874
www.doh.state.fl.us

Georgia Composite State Board of Medical Examiners
LaSharn Hughes, Executive Director
2 Peachtree Street, NW, 36th Floor
Atlanta, GA 30303
(404) 656-3913
Fax: (404) 656-9723
www.medicalboard.state.ga.us

Guam Board of Medical Examiners
Chalsea Torres, Acting Administrator
Health Professionals Licensing Office
651 Legacy Square Commercial Complex
South Route 10, Ste. 9
Margilao, GU 96913
(011) 671-735-7406-8
Fax: (011) 671-735-7413

Hawaii Board of Medical Examiners
Constance Cabral, Executive Officer
Department of Commerce & Consumer Affairs
P.O. Box 3469
Honolulu, HI 96813
(street address: 335 Merchant St., Room 301, 96813)
(808) 586-3000
Fax: (808) 586-2874
www.hawaii.gov/dcca/pvl

Idaho State Board of Medicine
Nancy Kerr, Executive Director
1755 Westgate Drive, Ste. 140
Boise, ID 83704
(208) 327-7000
Fax: (208) 327-7005
www.bom.state.id.us

Illinois Department of Financial and Professional Regulation
Division of Professional Regulation, Daniel E. Bluthardt, Acting Director, Chicago Office (disciplinary issues)
Doris Barnes, Disciplinary Board Liaison
James R. Thompson Center
100 W Randolph St., Ste. 9-300
Chicago, IL 60601
(312) 814-4500
Fax: (312) 814-1837
www.ildfpr.com

Illinois Department of Financial and Professional Regulation
Division of Professional Regulation, Daniel E. Bluthardt, Acting Director, Springfield Office (licensure issues)
Sandra Dunn, Licensure Manager
320 W. Washington St., 3rd Floor
Springfield, IL 62786
(217) 785-0800
Fax: (217) 524-2169
www.ildfpr.com

Indiana Health Professions Bureau
Michael Rinebold, Board Director
402 W. Washington St., Room 041
Indianapolis, IN 46204
(317) 234-2960
Fax: (317) 233-4236
www.in.gov/pla/bandc/mlbi/

Iowa State Board of Medical Examiners
Ann Mowery, Ph.D., Executive Director
400 Southwest Eighth Street, Ste. C
Des Moines, IA 50309-4686
(515) 281-5171
Fax: (515) 242-5908
www.docboard.org/ia/ia_home.htm

Kansas Board of Healing Arts
Lawrence Buening Jr., J.D., Executive Director
235 South Topeka Blvd.
Topeka, KS 66603-3068
(785) 296-7413
Fax: (785) 296-0852
www.ksbha.org

Kentucky Board of Medical Licensure
C. William Schmidt, Executive Director
Hurstbourne Office Park
310 Whittington Parkway, Ste. 1B
Louisville, KY 40222-4916
(502) 429-7150
Fax: (502) 429-7158
kbml.ky.gov

Louisiana State Board of Medical Examiners
John B. Bobear, M.D., Executive Director
P.O. Box 30250
New Orleans, LA 70190-0250
(street address: 630 Camp St., 70130)
(504) 568-6820
Fax: (504) 568-8893
www.lsbme.louisiana.gov/

Maine Board of Licensure in Medicine Randal C. Manning, Executive Director 137 State House Station (U.S. mail) Augusta, ME 04333 (207) 287-3601 Fax: (207) 287-6590 www.docboard.org/me/me_home.htm	Maine Board of Osteopathic Licensure Susan E. Strout, Executive Secretary 142 State House Station Augusta, ME 04333-0142 (207) 287-2480 Fax: (207) 287-3015 www.maine.gov/osteo/	Maryland Board of Physicians C. Irving Pinder, Executive Director P.O. Box 2571 Baltimore, MD 21215-0095 (street address: 4201 Patterson Ave., 3rd Floor, 21215) (410) 764-4777 Fax: (410) 358-2252 (800) 492-6836 mbp.state.md.us/
Massachusetts Board of Registration in Medicine Nancy Achin Audesse, Executive Director 560 Harrison Ave., Ste. G-4 Boston, MA 02118 (617) 654-9800 Fax: (617) 451-9568 (800) 377-0550 www.massmedboard.org	Michigan Board of Medicine Rae Ramsdell, Licensing Director P.O. Box 30670 Lansing, MI 48909-8170 (street address: 611 W. Ottawa St., 1st Floor, 48933) (517) 335-0918 Fax: (517) 373-2179 www.michigan.gov/mdch	Michigan Board of Osteopathic Medicine and Surgery Rae Ramsdell, Licensing Director P.O. Box 30670 Lansing, MI 48909-8170 (street address: 611 W. Ottawa St., 1st Floor, 48933) (517) 335-0918 Fax: (517) 373-2179 www.michigan.gov/mdch
Minnesota Board of Medical Practice Robert A. Leach, J.D., Executive Director University Park Plaza 2829 University Ave. SE, Ste. 500 Minneapolis, MN 55414-3246 (612) 617-2130 Fax: (612) 617-2166 Hearing impaired: 1-(800) 627-3529 www.bmp.state.mn.us	Mississippi State Board of Medical Licensure W. Joseph Burnett, M.D., Director 1867 Crane Ridge Drive, Ste. 200B Jackson, MS 39216 (601) 987-3079 Fax: (601) 987-4159 www.msbml.state.ms.us	Missouri State Board of Registration for the Healing Arts Tina M. Steinman, Executive Director 3605 Missouri Blvd. Jefferson City, MO 65109 (street address: 3605 Missouri Blvd.) (573) 751-0098 Fax: (573) 751-3166 www.pr.mo.gov/healingarts.asp
Montana Board of Medical Examiners Jeannie Worsech, Executive Director P.O. Box 200513 Helena, MT 59620-0513 (406) 841-2300 Fax: (406) 841-2363 www.medicalboard.mt.gov	Nebraska Board of Medicine and Surgery Health and Human Services Regulation and Licensure Credentialing Division Becky Wisell, Section Administrator P.O. Box 94986 Lincoln, NE 68509-4986 (402) 471-2133 Fax: (402) 471-3577 www.hhs.state.ne.us/	Nevada State Board of Medical Examiners Tony Clark, J.D., Executive Secretary 1105 Terminal Way, Ste. 301 Reno, NV 89502 (775) 688-2559 Fax: (775) 688-2321 www.medboard.nv.gov

Nevada State Board of Osteopathic Medicine Larry J. Tarno, D.O., Executive Director 860 E. Flamingo Rd., Ste. G Las Vegas, NV 89121 (702) 732-2147 Fax: (702) 732-2079 www.osteo.state.nv.us	New Hampshire Board of Medicine Penny Taylor, Administrator 2 Industrial Park Drive, Ste. 8 Concord, NH 03301-8520 (603) 271-1203 Fax: (603) 271-6702 Complaints: (800) 780-4757 www.state.nh.us/medicine	New Jersey State Board of Medical Examiners William V. Roeder, Executive Director P.O. Box 183 Trenton, NJ 08625-0183 (609) 826-7100 Fax: (609) 826-7117 www.state.nj.us/lps/ca/medical.htm#bme5
New Mexico Medical Board Charlotte Kinney, Executive Director 2055 S. Pacheco, Building 400 Santa Fe, NM 87505 (505) 476-7220 Fax: (505) 476-7237 www.state.nm.us/nmbme	New Mexico Board of Osteopathic Medical Examiners Annette Rodriguez Brumley, Executive Director 2550 Cerrillos Road Santa Fe, NM 87501-5101 (505) 476-4695 Fax: (505) 476-4665 www.rld.state.nm.us/b&c/Osteo	New York State Board for Medicine (Licensure) Thomas J. Monahan, Executive Secretary 89 Washington Avenue, 2nd Floor, West Wing Albany, NY 12234 (518) 474-3817 Ext. 560 Fax: (518) 486-4846 www.op.nysed.gov/proflist.htm
New York State Board for Professional Medical Conduct (Discipline) Dennis J. Graziano, Executive Director Department of Health Office of Professional Medical Conduct 433 River St., Ste. 303 Troy, NY 12180-2299 (518) 402-0855 Fax: (518) 402-0866 www.health.state.ny.us/nysdoh/opmc/	North Carolina Medical Board R. David Henderson, J.D., Executive Director P.O. Box 20007 Raleigh, NC 27619 (919) 326-1100 Fax: (919) 326-1130 www.ncmedboard.org	North Dakota State Board of Medical Examiners Rolf P. Sletten, J.D., Executive Secretary/Treasurer City Center Plaza 418 E. Broadway, Ste. 12 Bismarck, ND 58501 (701) 328-6500 Fax: (701) 328-6505 www.ndbomex.com
Northern Mariana Islands Medical Professional Licensing Board Juanet S. Crisostomo, Administrator P.O. Box 501458, CK Saipan, MP 96950 (670) 664-4811 Fax: (670) 664-4813	State Medical Board of Ohio Richard A. Whitehouse, Esq., Executive Director 77 S. High St., 17th Floor Columbus, OH 43215-6127 (614) 466-3934 Fax: (614) 728-5946 (800) 554-7717 www.med.ohio.gov	Oklahoma State Board of Medical Licensure and Supervision Lyle Kelsey, C.A.E., Executive Director P.O. Box 18256 Oklahoma City, OK 73118 (405) 848-6841 Fax: (405) 848-8240 (800) 381-4519 www.okmedicalboard.org

Oklahoma State Board of
Osteopathic Examiners
Gary R. Clark, Executive Director
4848 N. Lincoln Blvd, Ste. 100
Oklahoma City, OK 73105-3321
(405) 528-8625
Fax: (405) 557-0653
www.okmedicalboard.org

Oregon Board of Medical
Examiners
Kathleen Haley, J.D., Executive
Director
1500 SW First Avenue, 620
Crown Plaza
Portland, OR 97201-5826
(503) 229-5770
Fax: (503) 229-6543
www.bme.state.or.us

Pennsylvania State Board of
Medicine
Joanne Troutman, Administrator
P.O. Box 2649
Harrisburg, PA 17105-2649
(717) 787-2381
Fax: (717) 787-7769
www.dos.state.pa.us

Pennsylvania State Board of
Osteopathic Medicine
Gina K. Bittner, Administrator
P.O. Box 2649
Harrisburg, PA 17105-2649
(street address: 124 Pine St.,
17101)
(717) 783-4858
Fax: (717) 787-7769
www.dos.state.pa.us

Board of Medical Examiners of
Puerto Rico
Pablo Valentin-Torres, Esq.,
Executive Director
P.O. Box 13969
San Juan, PR 00908
(787) 792-8949
Fax: (787) 792-4436

Rhode Island Board of Medical
Licensure and Discipline
Robert S. Crausman, M.D., Chief
Administrator
Department of Health
Cannon Building, Room 205
Three Capitol Hill
Providence, RI 02908-5097
(401) 222-3855
Fax: (401) 222-2158
www.health.ri.gov/hsr/bmld/

South Carolina Board of Medical
Examiners
Department of Labor, Licensing
and Regulation
John D. Volmer, Board
Administrator
110 Centerview Drive, Ste. 202
Columbia, SC 29210-1289
(803) 896-4500
Fax: (803) 896-4515
www.llr.state.sc.us/pol/medical

South Dakota State Board
of Medical and Osteopathic
Examiners
L. Paul Jensen, Executive
Secretary
1323 S. Minnesota Ave.
Sioux Falls, SD 57105
(605) 334-8343
Fax: (605) 336-0270
www.state.sd.us/dcr/medical

Tennessee Board of Medical
Examiners
Rosemarie Otto, Executive
Director
425 5th Ave. North, 1st Floor,
Cordell Hull Building
Nashville, TN 37247-1010
(615) 532-3202
Fax: (615) 253-4484
www.state.tn.us/health

Tennessee Board of Osteopathic
Examiners
Rosemarie Otto, Executive
Director
425 5th Ave. North, 1st Floor,
Cordell Hull Building
Nashville, TN 37247-1010
(615) 532-3202
Fax: (615) 253-4484
Toll-free: (888) 310-4650
www.state.tn.us/health

Texas State Board of Medical
Examiners
Donald W. Patrick, M.D., J.D.,
Executive Director
P.O. Box 2018
Austin, TX 78768-2018
(512) 305-7010
Fax: (512) 305-7008
Disciplinary Hotline:
(800) 248-4062
Consumer Complaint Hotline:
(800) 201-9353
www.tsbme.state.tx.us

Utah Department of Commerce
Div. of Occupational &
Professional Licensure
Physicians Licensing Board
Craig J. Jackson, R.Ph.
160 E 300 South, 84102, Heber
M. Wells Building, 4th Floor
Salt Lake City, UT 84114
(801) 530-6628
Fax: (801) 530-6511
www.dopl.utah.gov

Utah Department of Commerce
Div. of Occupational &
Professional Licensure
Board of Osteopathic Medicine
Diana T. Baker, Bureau Manager
160 E 300 South, 84102, Heber
M. Wells Building, 4th Floor
Salt Lake City, UT 84114
(801) 530-6628
Fax: (801) 530-6511
www.dopl.utah.gov

Vermont Board of Medical
Practice
Paula DiStabile, Executive
Director
108 Cherry Street
Burlington, VT 05402-0070
(802) 657-4220
Fax: (802) 657-4227
www.healthvermont.gov/hc/
med_board/profiles.aspx

Vermont Board of Osteopathic
Physicians and Surgeons
Jessica Porter, Director, Office of
Professional Regulation
26 Terrace Street, Drawer 09
Montpelier, VT 05609-1106
(802) 828-2373
Fax: (802) 828-2465
www.vtprofessionals.org

Virgin Islands Board of Medical
Examiners
Lydia Scott, Executive Assistant
Department of Health
48 Sugar Estate
St. Thomas, VI 00802
(340) 774-0117
Fax: (340) 777-4001

Virginia Board of Medicine
William L. Harp, M.D., Executive
Director
6603 W. Broad St., 5th Floor
Richmond, VA 23230-1717
(804) 662-9908
Fax: (804) 662-9517
www.vahealthprovider.com

Washington Medical Quality
Assurance Commission
Blake T. Maresh, M.P.A.,
Executive Director
Department of Health
310 Israel Road, SE
MS 47866
Tumwater, WA 98501
(360) 236-4788
Fax: (360) 586-4573
www.doh.wa.gov

Washington State Board of
Osteopathic Medicine and
Surgery
Blake Maresh, Executive Director
Department of Health
P.O Box 47866
Olympia, WA 98504-7866
(360) 236-4945
Fax: (360) 236-2406
www.doh.wa.gov

West Virginia Board of Medicine
101 Dee Drive
Charleston, WV 25311
(304) 558-2921
Fax: (304) 558-2084
www.wvdhhr.org/wvbom

West Virginia Board of
Osteopathy
Cheryl Schreiber, Executive
Secretary
334 Penco Rd.
Weirton, WV 26062
(304) 723-4638
Fax: (304) 723-2877
www.wvbdosteo.org

Wisconsin Medical Examining
Board
Department of Regulation and
Licensing
Thomas Ryan, Bureau Director
1400 E. Washington Ave.
Madison, WI 53703
(608) 266-2112
Fax: (608) 261-7083
www.drl.state.wi.us

Wyoming Board of Medicine
Carole Shotwell, J.D., Executive
Secretary
211 W. 19th St., Colony Bldg.,
2nd Floor
Cheyenne, WY 82002
(307) 778-7053
Fax: (307) 778-2069
wyomedboard.state.wy.us/
roster.asp

Glossary

— — — — — — — — — — — — — — — — — — — —

access: The process or system by which care is dispensed.

advocate: A person who supports or defends.

Annual health care liability: The approximate budgeted potential cost a patient would incur in the event that a health care crisis arose and the patient were liable for all out-of-pocket and deductible limits in one benefit year.

apprehension index: A graph used to measure a patient's apprehension, anxiety, or stress as it relates to the patient's care experience while interacting with a health care system.

billed charge: The retail price for procedure(s) or service(s).

certificate of coverage: A legal document provided to the group member from the insurance company describing the general policy provisions for eligibility, deductibles, coinsurance, maximums, and benefits covered, and so on.

Children's Health Insurance Program (CHIP): The federal-state Children's Health Insurance Program (CHIP), created under the new Title XXI of the Social Security Act. The program provides health coverage to uninsured children whose families earn too much for Medicaid but too little to afford private coverage. For more information, go to www.cms.gov.

CHIP: *See* Children's Health Insurance Program.

coinsurance: A patient's owed amount for services in addition to a plan's deductibles and co-payments. Coinsurance only applies to services covered by your health insurance.

contractual adjustment: If a provider or facility has a contract with an insurance company, the terms of the contract may stipulate that the provider or facility must discount billed charges in exchange for increased patient volume. The contractual adjustment represents the sum of money the provider or facility is obliged to reduce the billed charge per the terms of the contract.

co-payment: Co-pay pertains to a portion of the bill for which the patient is responsible, provided the service is covered by your plan.

cumulative lost lifetime: The amount of time lost participating in redundant tasks or inefficient systems that do not relate to healing or wellness over an extended period of time.

deductible: Provided services are covered by your plan, deductible is the patient's financial responsibility for all care and services rendered. Insurance begins paying for services once the deductible has been reached. Each new plan year typically has a deductible.

Department of Health and Human Services: The Department of Health and Human Services is the U.S. government's principal agency for protecting the health of all Americans and providing essential human services, especially for those who are least able to help themselves.

D.O.: *See* Doctor of Osteopathy.

Doctor of Osteopathy (D.O.): A doctor who practices osteopathic medicine. *See* osteopathic medicine.

Doctor of Philosophy (Ph.D.): The highest academic degree awarded by a university to students who have completed studies beyond the bachelor's and/or master's degrees, and who have demonstrated their academic ability in oral and written examinations and through original research presented in the form of a dissertation (thesis).

EAP: *See* Employee Assistance Program.

eligible expenses: A term usually found in language relating to insurance coverage. The term refers to the portion of a provider's billed charge that is eligible for reimbursement under the terms of the agreement between the patient and the provider.

Employee Assistance Program (EAP): An employer-sponsored benefit that offers work-life balance support to employees and their family members.

EOB: *See* explanation of benefits.

exclusions: Services not covered by insurance.

exclusions database: The exclusions database, administered by the Office of Inspector General and available at www.oig.hhs.gov/fraud/exclusions.html, tracks providers who are ineligible to receive payment from federal health care programs.

experimental: Medical, surgical, diagnostic, psychiatric, substance abuse, or other health care services, technologies, supplies, treatments, procedures, drug therapies, or devices that, at the time the insurance company makes its determination regarding coverage, are generally treatments not approved by the U.S. Food and Drug Administration (FDA), or services not identified by the American Hospital Formulary Service or the United States Pharmacopoeia Dispensing Information as appropriate for use. A patient's certificate of coverage should outline what determines experimental or investigational services.

explanation of benefits (EOB): A document produced by the insurance company outlining the benefit coverage of services rendered. The document typically outlines what the insurance company pays for the service(s) and what portion is the patient's responsibility. This document is also referred to as a remittance advice, or RA.

facility: A hospital, emergency clinic, outpatient clinic, or other entity providing health care as credentialed by Centers for Medicare and Medicaid Services.

federal health care program: Health care programs funded by the federal government. Medicare, Medicaid, and Children's Health Insurance Program (CHIP) are examples of federal health care programs.

fellowship: A period of training for physicians, usually one to two years, that occurs after completion of a general or primary residency. Its goal is to qualify a physician as a subspecialist in an area of medical practice such as cardiology, hand surgery, or other specialty.

Flex spend account (FSA): An employer-sponsored account funded by the employee for medical expenses not covered by the employee's insurance. The funds contributed to the account are tax free to the employee. Funds remaining in the account at the end of the plan year are forfeited.

glioblastoma multiforme: A type of brain tumor that forms from glial (supportive) tissue of the brain. It grows very quickly and has cells that look very different from normal cells. Also called grade IV astrocytoma.

guarantor: The person responsible for paying the patient's bill.

health insurance: An insurance policy that will pay for certain medical treatments or services.

health insurance premium: *See* premium.

Health Plan Employers Data and Information Set (HEDIS): HEDIS is a set of standardized performance measures designed to ensure that purchasers and consumers have the information they need to reliably compare the performance of managed health care plans. The performance measures in HEDIS are related to many significant public health issues such as cancer, heart disease, smoking, asthma, and diabetes. HEDIS also includes a standardized survey of consumer's experiences that evaluates plan performance in areas such as customer service, access to care, and claims possessing. HEDIS is sponsored, supported, and maintained by NCQA.

health savings account (HSA): An HSA is a tax-exempt trust or custodial account that you set up with a qualified HSA trustee to pay or reimburse certain medical expenses you incur. You must be an eligible individual to qualify for an HSA account. The funds deposited are tax exempt.

HEDIS: *See* Health Plan Employers Data and Information Set.

hospital inpatient: When a person is admitted to a hospital for more than twenty-four hours, the visit is considered an inpatient visit. Generally, the facility is providing room and board in addition to health-related services.

in-network: Insurance companies build networks of providers and facilities. The concept of in-network means there is a contractual agreement between the provider or facility and the insurance company. To be deemed in-network is to be engaged in a contractual agreement with an insurance company.

inpatient: A patient who is formally admitted to a facility and typically stays in the facility longer than twenty-four hours. Generally, the facility is providing room and board in addition to health-related services.

insurance claim: Demand for payment in accordance with an insurance policy. The information necessary for a patient's health insurance experience to be considered and possibly paid by the insurance covering the patient.

internship: A period of apprenticeship when medical students work off-campus, under supervision, typically in a hospital. It allows students to learn practical applications of classroom material.

investigational: *See* experimental.

Joint Commission on Accreditation of Healthcare Organizations (JCAHO): The organization's mission is to continuously improve the safety and quality of care provided to the public through the provision of health care accreditation and related services that support performance improvement in health care organizations.

licensure: Legal permission granted by a state or territorial government to a physician to take personal, unsupervised responsibility for the diagnosis and treatment of patients in the practice of medicine. Most states and territories require that physicians complete at least one year, and several require three years, of graduate medical education to qualify for licensure. In addition, applicants for licensure must pass an examination. Qualifications for medical licensure in each jurisdiction are determined by that jurisdiction. Federal, state, and territorial governments do not license physicians as specialists, nor certify physicians as specialists.

lost lifetime: The amount of time lost participating in redundant or inefficient systems or tasks that do not relate to healing or wellness.

M.D.: *See* medical doctor.

maximum policy benefit: The greatest amount the insurance company will pay for services covered by the plan.

Medicaid: A program sponsored by the federal government and administered by states that is intended to provide health care and health-related services to low-income individuals.

medical doctor: A doctorate-level degree held by people who are medical doctors (M.D.s).

Medicare: A federal health insurance program for people age sixty-five and older and for individuals with disabilities.

National Association of Insurance Commissioners (NAIC): The mission of the NAIC is to assist state insurance regulators, individually and collectively, in serving the public interest and achieving the following fundamental insurance regulatory goals in a responsive, efficient, and cost-effective manner, consistent with the wishes of its members: protect the public interest; promote competitive markets; facilitate the fair and equitable treatment of insurance consumers; promote the reliability, solvency, and financial solidity of insurance institutions; and support and improve state regulation of insurance.

National Committee for Quality Assurance (NCQA): The organization's mission is to improve the quality of health care through measurement, transparency, and accountability. The committee's core values are improving the quality of health care, standing for accountability throughout the health care system, providing information to empower people to make informed decisions, and providing excellent customer service.

network: Insurance companies create networks of providers for the purpose of controlling costs and ensuring comprehensive patient care. Providers in the network have a contract with the insurance company generally to see the patients insured by the insurance company at a reduced reimbursement.

noncovered services: Health-related procedures, supplies, and services not reimbursed by the patient's insurance policy.

Office of Inspector General (OIG): The mission of the Office of Inspector General, as mandated by Public Law 95-452 (as amended), is to protect the integrity of Department of Health and Human Services (HHS) programs, as well as the health and welfare of the beneficiaries of those programs. The OIG reports both to the HHS secretary and to the Congress, informing them of program and management problems and makes recommendations to correct them. The OIG's duties are carried out through a nationwide network of audits, investigations, inspections, and other mission-related functions performed by OIG components.

osteopathic medicine: Osteopathic medicine is a system of health care based on the premise that disease is the result of the relationship between anatomical structure and physiological function. Structure and function are considered interdependent and a normally functioning musculoskeletal system plays an important role in wellness, disease prevention, and recovery. Osteopathic physicians may use all accepted medical means including surgery, drugs, patient education, and manipulation of the body.

out-of-network benefits: The benefits provided by a patient's insurance coverage when the patient receives care outside the defined network, as stipulated by the insurance company.

out-of-pocket maximum: The maximum or limit to the patient's annual cost for health care services *covered* by the patient's health insurance.

outpatient: A patient who utilizes the services of a hospital or inpatient facility but is not formally admitted to the facility and typically does not remain at the facility for more than twenty-four hours.

patient advocate: A person who facilitates communication between a patient and his or her caregivers. The patient advocate focuses on creating the experience the patient desires.

personal health record: A patient's comprehensive record of his or her health and health care experiences, providers, facilities, contacts, medications, allergies, and services.

Ph.D.: *See* doctor of philosophy.

physician services: Procedures performed or services provided by medical doctors (M.D.s) or doctors of osteopathy (D.O.s).

preauthorization: *See* precertification.

precertification: Precertification, or preauthorization, is an insurance company's mechanism to control costs and to be aware of the services your physician is recommending for your treatment plan.

preexisting condition: Taken literally, a physical or health-related condition in existence prior to the effective date of insurance policy coverage. A patient subscribing to new health benefits with established need for care (in other words, a patient with a current health condition requiring care) who is beginning a new health insurance plan. The plan may have language excluding or limiting reimbursement for such situations.

premium: The cost to purchase insurance.

provider: Any person or organization that provides medical or health services, bills for them, and is paid for them.

RA: *See* explanation of benefits.

reimbursement: To repay or make restoration of equivalent value.

remittance advice (RA): *See* explanation of benefits.

residency: A medical residency is a postgraduate educational and clinical training program for physicians in the United States of America. It is filled by a resident physician who has received a postgraduate medical degree (M.D. or D.O.) and is enrolled in a clinical training program, generally affiliated with a hospital.

SOAP note: The acronym SOAP stands for Subjective, Objective, Assessment, and Plan. In a clinical setting, it offers structure to a patient's clinical treatment plan and record. In a patient's self-maintained medical record, it offers the same structure, but from the patient's perspective instead of the clinician's perspective.

specialty: The doctor's specialty is the sector of medicine the person practices. Doctor's can have more than one specialty or subspecialty. For example, a doctor caring for young children is a pediatric physician, and pediatrics is his or her specialty. A doctor whose care focuses on performing surgery for young children is a pediatric surgeon, and that is his or her subspecialty.

State Board of Medical Examiners: The state entity responsible for licensure of medical doctors or doctors of osteopathy.

subscriber: The person who holds or purchases the health insurance policy and is named in the certificate of coverage.

subspecialty: A subspecialty is a more focused or defined practice of care. It is a subset of a broader branch of medicine. If surgery is a specialty, then cardiothoracic surgery is a subspecialty of surgery.

temporomandibular joint dysfunction: A painful condition involving the temporomandibular joint and the muscles used for chewing. The condition sometimes causes clicking sounds and restricted jaw movement. It is a common and sometimes overlooked cause of chronic headaches.

TMJ: *See* temporomandibular joint dysfunction.

underinsured: A patient with health insurance who cannot afford the health-related costs associated with care not covered by his or her health insurance.

uninsured: A patient with no health insurance.

Endnotes

1. Keenan, John; "Review of SOAP Note Charting," Department of Family Medicine, www.meded.umn.edu, August 16, 2006.
2. Unitedhealthcare Choice, *Certificate of Coverage*, January 2005.
3. Ibid.
4. Unitedhealthcare Choice Plus, *Certificate of Coverage*, January 2005.
5. Keenan, "Review of SOAP."

Index
